Praise for
Before the Scalpel:
What Everyone Should Know about Anesthesia

"Dr. Dhar's book is so readable, concise, and informative that it should be assigned reading by surgeons and physicians to their patients who are preparing for surgery or procedures requiring sedation. *Before the Scalpel* reaches a difficult balance by being substantive enough to provide a review for the medical professional while being easily comprehensible to the layperson. Very timely publication; it fills that . . . gap in every patient's operative preparation."

—Robert M. Rey, MD, MPP, featured on E! Entertainment's hit series *Dr. 90210*

"The book is beautifully written in a simple yet elegant style, presenting extremely difficult concepts in an easy-to-understand format. . . . Every sentence, every concept is crisp and concise and valuable to anyone who plans an operating room experience. . . . All surgeons should make this book available to their patients to read."

—Ira H. Kirschenbaum, MD, founding executive director of Medscape Orthopaedics, now part of the WebMD family

"In an age of information overload, anesthesia—the 'art of comfort'—remains the dark continent of medicine for most patients. We put ourselves in the presiding doctor's hands blindly, trusting that our pain and awareness will be dulled in exchange for giving ourselves over to the needle, the gas mask, the IV full of narcotics and sedatives. *Before the Scalpel* does an admirable job of closing this gap, presenting the whys and wherefores of anesthesia in a crisp and lucid style. Panchali Dhar has thought of all the possible questions and fears that patients might have concerning this crucial but mostly unexplained procedure and addresses them one by one. This is a must-read for anyone who wants to be better informed about his or her medical care."

—Daphne Merkin, novelist, critic, and contributing writer to *The New York Times Magazine*

"Dr. Dhar's book is a welcome 'first of its kind' in helping patients understand and demystify the process of having major surgery."

—Richard Lavely, MD, JD, MS, MPH, Yale University School of Medicine and Yale School of Public Health

"A must-read for all of us who fear undergoing anesthesia. Dr. Dhar provides reassurance with her detailed but easily understandable explanations of the anesthesia process before, during, and after surgery. By imparting her knowledge and sage advice, she helps patients become enlightened and empowered to help themselves in a situation that often requires relinquishing control of consciousness. . . . Kudos to Dr. Dhar for making the complicated world of anesthesia so comprehensible!"
—Lisa G. Newman, MD, assistant professor of medicine, NYU School of Medicine

"Dr. Panchali Dhar sends a clear message essential to the most important tenet we all seek: patient safety through education, which leads to knowledge, which leads to empowerment."
—Carol Weihrer, The Anesthesia Awareness Campaign

"In *Before the Scalpel*, [Panchali Dhar] has given us the right information, at the right time, and presented the right way. Perfect! All my patients, family, and friends having surgeries will be getting a copy!"
—Rodney Dunetz, MS, AP, DOM, acupuncture physician and doctor of oriental medicine, Boca Raton, FL

"*Before the Scalpel* is an impressively thorough, informative, educational, concise, and demystifying reference guide for the emotionally unprepared surgical patient, in addition to any and all health care professionals involved with the surgical process."
—Thomas Bolte, MD, medical director of Bolte Medical, New York City

wishing you
good health
and sweet dreams
Panchali Dhar

before
the
scalpel

{ what everyone
should
know about
anesthesia

Panchali Dhar, MD

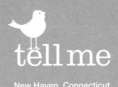

tell me

New Haven, Connecticut

Great care has been taken to ensure the accuracy of the information presented in this book and to describe generally accepted medical practices. The author, editors, and publisher are not responsible for errors or omissions or for any application of the information in this book and make no warranty, either implied or expressed, with regard to this edition or future editions of the content of this book.

Photo credits: Cartoonstock: pp 32, 41, 104 (bottom). Panchali Dhar: pp 11, 124 (top), 150. Getty Images: front cover. iStockphoto: pp 3, 5 (top), 8–9, 16–19, 23, 25–26, 33 (mask, sleeper), 44, 45 (bottom), 52–53, 55 (bottom), 56–57, 61–63, 75–76, 79–80, 82, 85, 87, 89–90, 92, 98–99, 104 (top), 105–106, 107 (left), 108, 111, 116, 119, 120, 122 (bottom), 124 (left), 128, 134, 138–139, 147, 149–150, 152–154, 157, 160, 162–164, 167, 169, 172–173, 179–181. Jupiterimages: p 137. Patricia A. Kuharic: pp 7, 33 (two hands), 35, 45 (top), 55 (top), 58, 83, 93, 113, 129, 143, 151, 161, 171. Torrie Lloyd-Masters: pp 140–141. Shutterstock: pp 5 (bottom), 15, 29, 33 (doctor, clock), 39–40, 49, 51, 64, 77, 103, 107 (right), 115, 122 (top), 127, 142. Patrick Timlin: pp 131–132.

Wong-Baker FACES Pain Rating Scale (p 88): from Hockenberry MJ, Wilson D, Winkelstein ML: *Wong's Essentials of Pediatric Nursing*, ed. 7, St. Louis, 2005, p 1259. Used with permission. Copyright, Mosby.

ISBN-13: 978-0-9816453-0-8

Library of Congress Control Number: 2008910756

Printed in the United States of America
First Edition January 2009
10 9 8 7 6 5 4 3 2 1

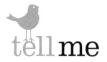

Published by Tell Me Press
98 Mansfield St.
New Haven, CT 06511
www.tellmepress.com

Editorial director: Lisa Clyde Nielsen
Managing editor: Paula Brisco
Text and cover designer: Linda Loiewski
Print production: Jeff Eyrich, Ian A. Nielsen, Jeff Breuler
Art program: Linda Loiewski
Editors: Paula Brisco, Laura Daly, Mimi Egan
Proofreaders: Roberta Monaco, Heather Carreiro
Indexer: Michael Monaco

contents

acknowledgments

Sincere thanks go to the people who inspired and encouraged me early in the project and beyond, including Dr. Gary Alevy and his wife, Denise; Jim and Beth Lewis; and Lisa and Ian Nielsen of Tell Me Press. Lisa and Ian have been pillars of support in making this book a reality. Their faith in me has been nothing less than energizing.

I would also like to express my appreciation to the publishing, design, marketing, and PR whizzes who have taught me so much about making books: Paula Brisco, Linda Loiewski, Jeff Eyrich, and Gail Parenteau of Parenteau Guidance.

Many colleagues and friends have given me countless suggestions and editorial insights: Farida Gadalla, MD; Susan Fagiani, RN; Gregory Kerr, MD; Sharon Abramowitz, MD; Miles Dinner, MD; Peter Goldstein, MD; David Behrman, DMD; Keith Lustman, DMD; Lisa Nigro, CRNA; Kevin de la Roza, MD; Abiona Berkeley, MD; Jon Samuels, MD; Patricia Mack, MD; and Patricia Kuharic, RBP.

I must mention the moral support and encouragement that I continually receive from Keisha Brown; Kathleen Burke, RN; Vinod Malhotra, MD; Ralph Slepian, MD; Thomas J. Fahey III, MD; Maamoun Jabali, MD; Natalia Ivascu, MD; Judith Weingram, MD; Carol Klein, CRNA; Rick Fuhry; Roberta Kirschenbaum; and my parents, Bani and Amiya.

Finally, special thanks must be extended to the Department of Anesthesiology at New York-Presbyterian Hospital, Weill Cornell Medical College of Cornell University for the opportunity to practice and foster relationships in the cutting-edge place it is.

introduction

More than seventy million Americans undergo surgical procedures every year. By age fifty, the average person has already had at least three surgeries requiring anesthesia.

Don't believe me?

Think about it—even if you haven't stepped foot in a hospital since you were born, you might have had your wisdom teeth removed by a dentist, a pesky mole whisked away by a dermatologist, or a broken arm set by a surgeon.

When a scalpel is involved, some form of anesthesia will be used. Anesthesia is also a part of diagnostic medical procedures that don't involve an incision. Anesthesia makes people comfortable while undergoing surgery and diagnostic procedures.

It is important to understand the anesthetic process; otherwise, you may find yourself in the backseat of your medical care. My goal is to empower you to sit in the front seat of your care.

We have all heard stories of things going catastrophically wrong during or after the time of surgical procedures—such as what occurred to author Olivia Goldsmith and to Donda West, the mother of musician Kanye West. Both women died, and the circumstances surrounding their deaths raised questions in our minds about the safety of surgery and anesthesia. These cases encourage us to learn more about the many factors that affect our medical care.

Then there are those frightening stories of people who were awake and aware during an operation—when their doctors believed they were unconscious.

These cases are few and far between, but they certainly make us think about something awful happening to us or someone we love.

Like most people, you probably have many questions about anesthesia. Everyone knows what the surgeon does, but what about the anesthesia providers? Who are they? What do they do after putting you to sleep or sedating you? How vital is their work?

The public perception of anesthesiologists is of doctors who do something really important, but the details of their work are usually vague. The word "anesthesia" evokes both a sense of comfort (as you are relieved to know you won't feel pain during surgery) and of fear (as you worry about the possibility that something can go wrong). Where can you learn to empower yourself and ask the right questions? The answers are in this book.

Before the Scalpel: What Everyone Should Know about Anesthesia is designed to help you, your friends, and your loved ones learn about anesthetic options and make more educated decisions. It will help you understand what anesthetic approaches are available today and which one is right for you. After all, there is no cookie-cutter or one-size-fits-all anesthetic that can be applied to everyone. Your medical history, body shape and size, physical health, and emotional needs are factors that must be taken into account when selecting a type of anesthetic.

> *As you read this book, watch for alert icons on the page: they flag issues that directly affect your anesthetic care. In addition, you'll find sidebars that emphasize topics relevant to your health and words in boldface that highlight equipment, techniques, and medical jargon to take the mystery out of medical practice. Most important, each chapter ends with a checklist of "prescriptives" that you can go through to make sure you receive the best care from doctors. Take this book with you to your doctor's office so you can ask the right questions and properly prepare for your medical procedure or surgery.*

Science is advancing rapidly. New medical breakthroughs are improving our lives in ways small and large and helping us live longer. Your informed knowledge of medical care today can increase the likelihood of your getting the most appropriate and comprehensive care available.

Toward that end, *Before the Scalpel: What Everyone Should Know about Anesthesia* is organized into four sections.

The first section, Anesthesia: The Art of Comfort, covers the people who make up your anesthesia providers—the A Team. These highly educated and experienced professionals work with your surgeon's team to bring you safely and comfortably through an operation or other medical procedure.

The second section of the book, It's Showtime! What to Expect, delves into the surgical experience itself, from pre-operative preparation through recovery. Your anesthesia providers are actively involved in caring for you during every part of this journey. You'll learn about what you can expect to experience before, during, and after surgery or another medical procedure. To give you reasons to feel more secure about your medical care, this section includes concrete descriptions of the protocols in place to protect you and details about how both your anesthesia providers and modern technology keep an eye on you.

The third section, Special Topics, addresses some of the most common medical circumstances that people experience. From choosing to undergo cosmetic surgery to controlling labor pain, from preparing for oral/dental surgery to readying your child for an operation, the common element is the use of anesthesia. You'll learn how anesthesiologists and other highly qualified anesthesia providers help you before, during, and after the Big Event to keep you and your loved ones safe and sound.

The final section, References and Tools, summarizes the history of anesthesia, briefly describes the medications commonly used to deliver anesthesia, presents a glossary of important terms (noted in boldface throughout the chapters), lists important references you might want to explore, and concludes with an index that allows you to quickly access topics that interest you most.

Being informed about your medical care means being empowered. Let this book open a new door to the world of anesthesia—a world that holds a unique place in our lives.

Panchali Dhar, MD

anesthesia { the art
of comfort

CHAPTERONE

at the helm:
the anesthesiologist

Who is that masked person at the head of the operating table? A physician? A technician? A nurse? And what exactly is that person doing?

That's the **anesthesiologist**, the person who will give you medications so that you won't feel any discomfort or pain during your surgery or other medical procedure.

As a patient, you may have known your **surgeon** for weeks, even years. Yet you probably won't meet your anesthesiologist until the very day of surgery. You *select* your surgeon, but you are usually *assigned* an anesthesiologist.

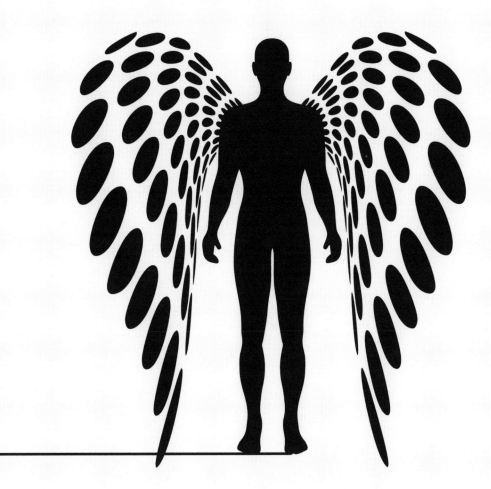

THINK OF THE ANESTHESIOLOGIST AS AN ANGEL WATCHING OVER YOU.

The anesthesiologist is at the helm in the operating room—working closely with the surgeon, monitoring the progress of the operation, and making sure you're safe while undergoing a surgery or procedure.

These days kids know the drill at the dentist's office, and lots of adults over age fifty know the routine of colonoscopy. But most people have no idea what an anesthesiologist actually does, besides the vague notion of "putting patients to sleep."

Anesthesia providers are responsible for your overall care just before, during, and after surgery. They are the ones who protect your health and safety during all types of procedures, from a deep cut made under general anesthesia—in which you are literally "put to sleep"—to a small nick that requires only local anesthesia to numb the area.

After reading this book, you will have a clearer idea of what's going on behind the scenes in the specialty of sleep and pain control. And you'll feel reassured knowing there's a highly qualified medical professional watching over you.

Meet the "A Team"

The A (as in anesthesia) Team includes **attending physician anesthesiologists, anesthesia residents, certified registered nurse anesthetists** (CRNAs), and **anesthesia assistants**.

The anesthesiologist is a physician, a highly trained doctor responsible for your well-being in the time surrounding your surgery. This is the person who monitors your heart rate, heart rhythm, breathing, oxygen level, blood pressure, pain level, anxiety level, movement, and **consciousness**. Anesthesiologists are the doctors who work behind the scenes and whom most patients don't remember—the doctors who keep you alive during the expected . . . and the unexpected.

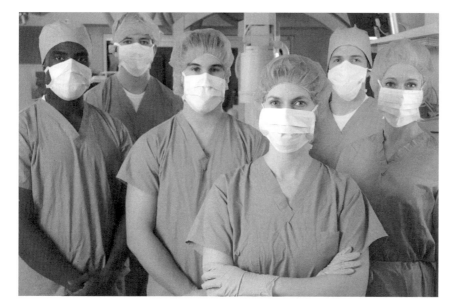

THE A TEAM

Many anesthesiologists work in surgeries related to their chosen field of expertise, such as cardiac, obstetric, neurosurgery, pediatric, orthopedic, thoracic, or vascular surgery. Some are involved in pain management. Today the anesthesiology specialty extends beyond the operating room. Anesthesiologists are also involved in intensive care units, trauma, pain relief for women in labor, and **sedation** of patients during **diagnostic procedures** such as colonoscopy, endoscopy, and magnetic resonance imaging (MRI).

In an average workday, the anesthesiologist applies knowledge of both medicine and surgery for the care of patients. An anesthesiologist, then, is a true **perioperative** physician—it's her job to address patient needs before, during, and after surgery.

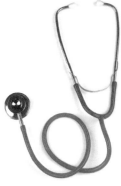

A physician anesthesia provider may be either a doctor still in training (a resident) or a fully trained attending physician. The typical anesthesia resident physician spends three years training in the specialty, after a preliminary year spent training in either internal medicine or surgery. You can rest assured—literally!—that anesthesia residents

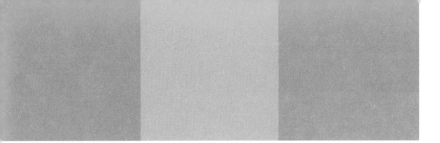

are perfectly qualified to handle your care. They have already completed years of specialized training. In addition, all residents work under the close supervision of an attending physician—the anesthesia provider who is ultimately responsible for your care.

 The attending anesthesiologist is present for all critical points in a case. She is always immediately available to "attend to" your needs. Sometimes the attending anesthesiologist supervises the care of two or three patients who are undergoing surgery at the same time in different operating rooms. In each room, the resident or CRNA is supervised by the attending anesthesiologist.

Training to be an anesthesiologist requires involvement in thousands of cases and meeting a certain, measurable level of competency. After training, the physician must take a standardized board-certification exam.

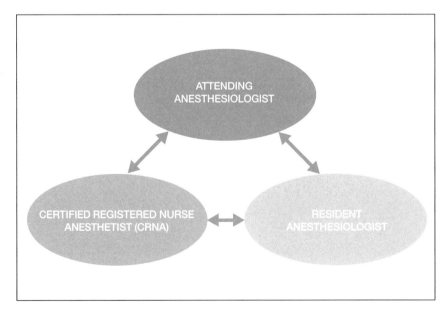

THE A TEAM PLAYERS WORK TOGETHER.

Once the physician passes, she is considered **board-certified**. This is a carefully verified level of professional achievement that recognizes consistency of both knowledge and training at a national level.

As a patient, you can always ask if the attending anesthesiologist is board-certified. A board-certified anesthesiologist is also required to participate in continuing education training each and every year.

A certified registered nurse anesthetist is often a part of the A Team. CRNAs usually work under the supervision of an attending anesthesiologist, but in some states they are permitted to work independently. They are fully qualified to deliver anesthesia for routine surgeries in hospitals and other settings.

Extensive training is required to become a CRNA. After graduating from a nursing program, a nurse must spend at least one year working in an intensive care setting, then she enters a specialized two-year anesthesia training program. She must pass a national certification program to become a CRNA and is encouraged to join the American Association of Nurse Anesthetists (AANA). A CRNA must also participate in continuing education programs each year.

PanchLines

Dr. Dhar Says: We Are Team Players

In this book, I sometimes use the term "anesthesia provider" to refer to either a fully trained physician anesthesiologist, a resident physician, or a certified registered nurse anesthetist. All of them completed rigorous training and had extensive hands-on experience before they were given the responsibility to oversee patients' lives during surgeries and other procedures.

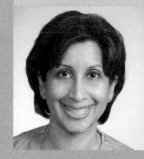

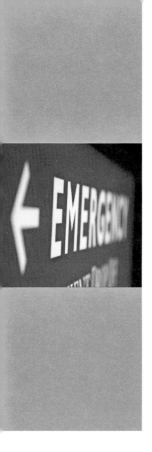

24/7 Care

Things can change very quickly during surgery. So in the world of anesthesia, there is no such thing as a typical day or a routine procedure. Every case is special and unique—just as you are.

Still, there are many constants in the anesthesiologist's workday, whether in a hospital or another medical setting.

An anesthesiologist may be asked to cover cases with residents and CRNAs in one, two, or even three operating rooms—all surgeries taking place at the same time. The daily schedule may change as emergency cases crop up and other surgeries are added. Of course, an emergency like acute appendicitis has to take precedence. Added cases may also take priority over scheduled ones. A member of the anesthesia team always reviews all available medical records before a patient enters the operating room.

If the anesthesiologist has specific concerns about a patient, she may ask the surgeon to order additional medical tests prior to **elective surgery** (a procedure that is not considered urgent, an emergency, or even medically necessary).

In emergencies, there may be no time for a leisurely conference. If your anesthesiologist has not met with you before you go in the operating room, or if you are unconscious when you enter the hospital, decisions have to be made quickly. But even emergency surgeries have an A Team to help you get through safely.

 No matter how short or long the surgery, at no time are you ever left without a qualified anesthesia provider at the head of the operating table.

In some cases, one attending anesthesiologist may transfer the care of a patient to another attending anesthesiologist. You may wake up after surgery and find a different person taking care of you. On occasion, the patient care is transferred from one anesthesia provider to another. Don't worry; you will never be left unattended. Your anesthesia provider may have been required to start another case, perhaps to help another anesthesiologist or go to an emergency in another part of the hospital. Meanwhile, another member of the A Team stepped in to care for you.

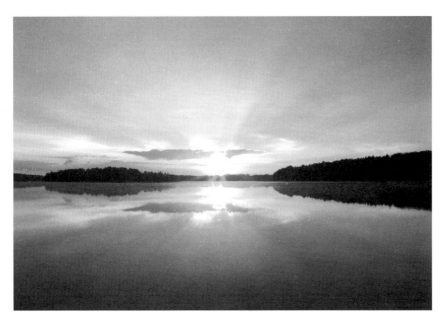

Sunrise, Sunset

Anesthesiologists are usually the first doctors to enter the hospital in the morning. They arrive at the crack of dawn. The first thing they do is set up the operating room to be ready for the patient. Then they activate the **anesthesia machine**—the staple, universal piece of equipment that defines their specialty. No other physician specialty knows how to work an anesthesia machine.

It's common for the A Team members to discuss the case before a surgery. During the discussion, they determine the **anesthetic plan**—a mental plan of what will be done for you before the scalpel. They may include the surgeon in the discussion if there are specific issues or surgical preferences. The anesthetic plan ensures that everyone is working together and with the same set of rules.

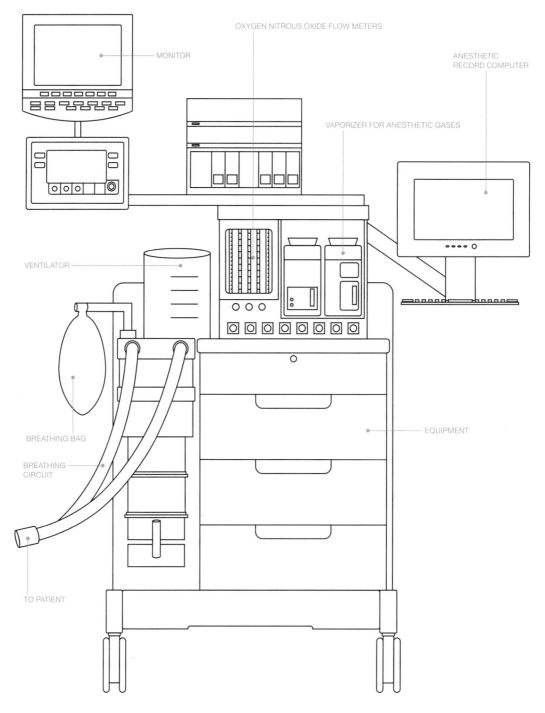

MONITOR

OXYGEN NITROUS OXIDE FLOW METERS

ANESTHETIC
RECORD COMPUTER

VAPORIZER FOR ANESTHETIC GASES

VENTILATOR

EQUIPMENT

BREATHING BAG

BREATHING
CIRCUIT

TO PATIENT

THE ANESTHESIA MACHINE: A MEDICAL WONDER THAT KEEPS YOU AT EASE!

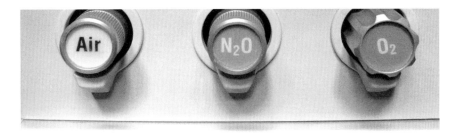

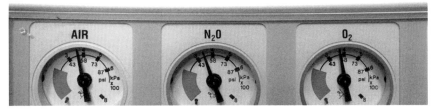

IMPORTANT ANESTHESIA GASES: AIR, NITROUS OXIDE (N₂O), AND OXYGEN (O₂)

> *The A Team welcomes your participation in making the anesthetic plan. As the patient, you may provide valuable insights—such as having a fear of needles, an addiction, or a family medical trait—that will lead to consideration of options to refine the anesthetic plan. We will talk extensively about your role in your anesthesia care in chapters 2 and 3.*

Every night in every hospital, an anesthesiologist or a team of anesthesia providers is **on-call**. In most hospitals the on-call professionals stay in the hospital to attend to any case that continues or arises during the night. Some hospitals permit the on-call professional to be available via beeper. And on weekends and holidays? There is always an anesthesia provider or team on-call to take care of you.

Off-Site Anesthesia

Anesthesia is not always confined to an operating room. A lot of nonsurgical and surgical procedures performed outside of the hospital's operating room require some type of anesthesia or sedation. Some of these procedures are done in **off-site locations**. These include imaging suites (such as for MRIs), cardiology catheterization labs, gastroenterology suites, intensive care units, emergency rooms, ophthalmology areas, and psychiatric treatment areas.

Anesthesia care also extends to non-hospital locations. An increasing number of medical procedures are done in **same-day** (or **ambulatory) surgery centers**, which (surprise!) are geared toward cases where patients are treated, then sent home the very same day. Examples of ambulatory surgeries are minor orthopedic cases, eye procedures, and many cosmetic surgeries. Other work sites are private doctors' offices where colonoscopies or endoscopies are done. These are called **office-based procedures**. It is growing as a field because more and more procedures are being done in non-hospital settings—including podiatry and dental offices. Another unique location is an **outpatient pain clinic** for treatment of chronic pain conditions (such as cancer pain and lower back pain).

The responsibility for ensuring safe anesthesia in *any* setting lies with the anesthesiologist. The equipment required for the delivery of safe patient care is always the same, and the same anesthesiology protocols still apply. For the anesthesiologist, this means having deep knowledge of the particular surgery, reviewing the patient's medical history, and seeing that all anesthesia equipment and medications are immediately available. The anesthesiologist's responsibility continues to caring for the patient immediately after surgery, and making sure they are on the safe road to recovery.

The Watchwords: Vigilance and Monitoring

Whether you're going under the scalpel or having a non-invasive procedure done, all eyes in the operating room are on the anesthesiologist to pull you through. And she will. Using sophisticated visual monitors, she is continuously watching your heart rate, heart rhythm, blood pressure, oxygen level, breathing, and other measures and indicators. Her job is not only about administering anesthesia and studying the monitors, it's also about watching what the surgeon is doing and supporting your life. All of this data is documented in what is the very important **anesthetic record**—an up-to-the-minute record of what is happening during surgery. It includes your **vital signs** (such as blood pressure and heart rate), medications given, and any events that occurred during the operation.

Vigilance and monitoring—and all the other tools and techniques she brings "to the table"—make the anesthesiologist the surgeon's partner in your medical care. Together, they and their teams steer you safely and comfortably through your procedure.

(Rx) **Prescriptives:** Be a Better Consumer

☐ **Who is providing your anesthetic care?** _____

_____

☐ **Is your care being directly provided by a doctor or nurse anesthetist?** _____

_____

☐ **Is the person providing your care board-certified?** _____

_____

☐ **What is the professional background of your anesthesia provider?** _____

_____

☐ **Where did your anesthesia provider get trained?** _____

_____

☐ **What is the location of your procedure?** _____

_____

☐ **A hospital operating room?** _____

_____

☐ **A location outside the hospital operating room?** _____

_____

☐ **An ambulatory surgery center?** _____

_____

☐ **A doctor's office?** _____

_____

choices, choices:
tools of the trade

Yes, as a patient you can be actively involved in making the anesthetic plan for your surgery or other medical procedure.

That said, not everyone has choices, because some operations can only be done with one type of anesthesia. For example, you won't be given a choice if you're having open-heart surgery. For that you'll need a general anesthetic.

The basic types of anesthesia—**local**, sedation with local (also known as **monitored anesthesia care**, or MAC), **regional**, and **general anesthesia**—have remained the

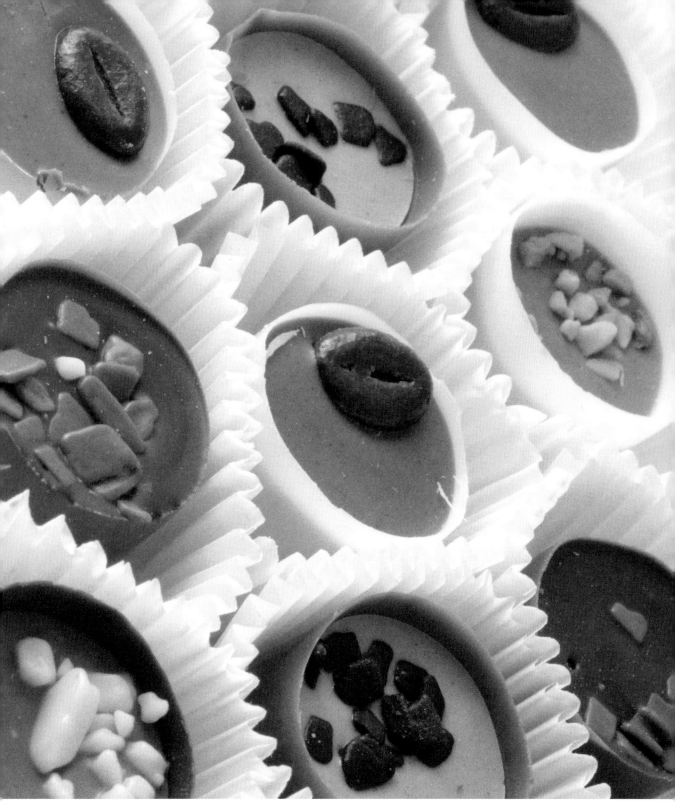

SOMETIMES THERE'S A CHOICE.

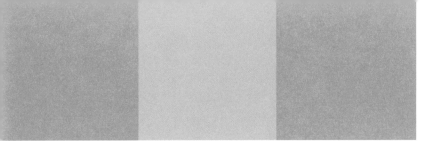

same for a century. What *is* evolving rapidly are the equipment, safety measures, modes of delivery, medications, and ease of application. Combined, the range of options allows the anesthesia provider to work more closely with you and help you make the best choice.

Not everyone wants to know everything about the surgery. In fact, some patients want to know as little as possible. They prefer to leave all decisions in the hands of their surgeon and anesthesiologist. But if you're the kind of person who likes to be in the know, the anesthesia provider will welcome your participation and desire to make an informed decision.

Let's go through the major types of anesthesia available today. We'll start with the simpler types and move on to the more complex.

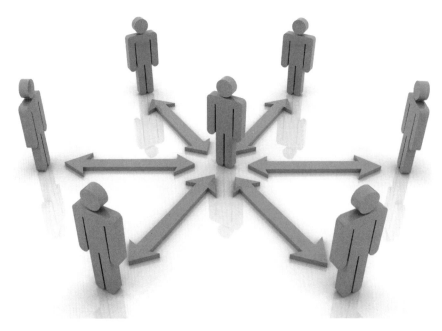

EVERYBODY HAS TO TALK TO THE ANESTHESIOLOGIST.

Everyone Is Different: The Physical Status Classification System

Anesthesiologists use a simple scoring system—the American Society of Anesthesiologists' (ASA) physical status score—to evaluate patients' health before they receive anesthesia. Patients are assigned a score from 1 to 6 based on their general health. The score does not depend on the type of surgery or the patient's age or gender.

The score is not a measure of risk, but studies have shown that it matches complications associated with surgery and anesthesia.

Overview of the ASA Physical Status Scoring System:*

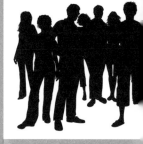

ASA 1: A normal, healthy patient

ASA 2: A patient with mild to moderate disease

ASA 3: A patient with severe disease that is not incapacitating

ASA 4: A patient with severe disease that is a constant threat to life

ASA 5: A patient who is not expected to survive without the operation

ASA 6: A declared brain-dead patient who is an organ donor

* The letter E is added after the number in cases of emergency surgery.

Numbing the Spot: Local Anesthesia

Suppose you're having surgery on a small area of your body, such as on your thumb, or you're having a few moles removed from your back. In these cases, the entire surrounding area doesn't need to be numbed, and you don't need to be put to sleep. Many short surgeries and diagnostic tests are done with a local anesthetic, which is a numbing medicine.

A popular term for local anesthetics is "novocaine," but there are many other types of local anesthetics. They vary in strength and duration of effect. When local anesthetics are injected around nerves in the area being worked on, pain signals from the nerves to the brain are blocked temporarily. A local anesthetic can be applied repeatedly in the same area, but with dosage limits.

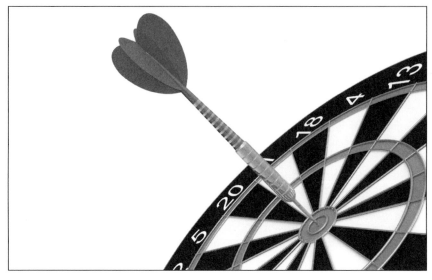

A LOCAL ANESTHETIC TARGETS A SPOT.

If a procedure is done as a "local," an anesthesiologist is not present. This usually implies that the surgery is minor and that the procedure will be brief. Local procedures are done in office settings and in hospitals. The doctor performing the procedure is the one who administers the local anesthetic. Many health-care professionals, such as surgeons, dermatologists, and dentists, are trained to inject local anesthetic in an office setting. For example, a dermatologist injects local anesthetic in an area of skin before taking a tissue sample (biopsy) to examine under a microscope.

The doctor performing the procedure may give the patient medication (oral or intravenous) to relax. In such circumstances, monitoring of blood pressure or oxygen level is recommended. A nurse or the doctor will follow up on the patient's proper recovery after the procedure.

It's Twilight Time: Monitored Anesthesia Care

The combination of undergoing surgery or a procedure and having an anesthesia provider present to deliver sedative medications is called monitored anesthesia care. It's also known as **twilight sleep**. Common surgeries done under MAC include hernia repair, eye, sinus, and certain

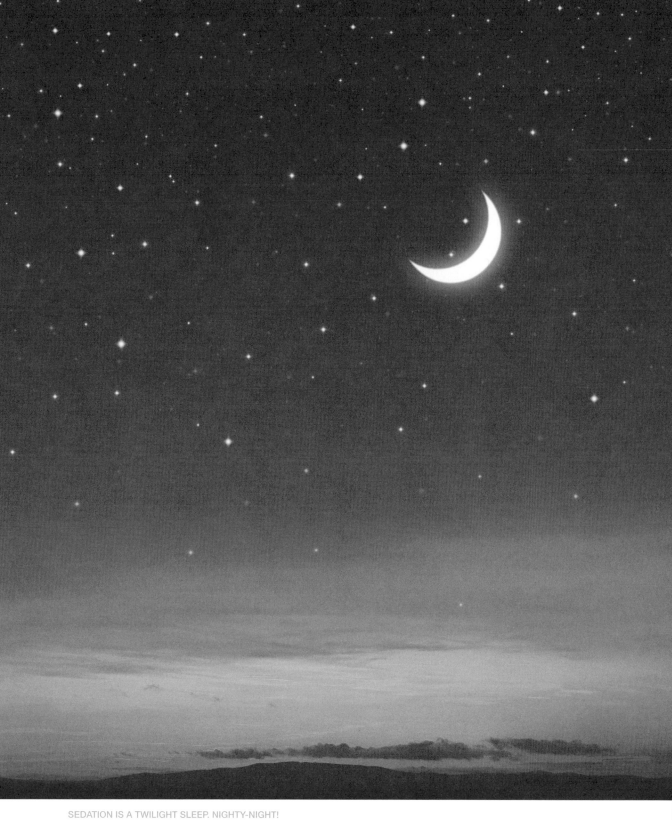

SEDATION IS A TWILIGHT SLEEP. NIGHTY-NIGHT!

plastic and vascular procedures. The most popular diagnostic procedures done in this manner are colonoscopy and endoscopy. The biopsy (sampling) of breast tissue to check for cancer is frequently done under MAC.

Many patients want to know exactly what MAC sedation means. Does it mean you will be awake? Does it mean you will hear everything being said in the room? Does it mean you will have to watch the procedure? The answer to all these questions is "no."

In certain MAC procedures, the surgeon applies local anesthetic around the part of the body being operated on. An anesthesiologist is always there to ensure your comfort and safety. The role of the anesthesiologist is to provide a mix of fast-acting and short-acting sedative drugs. The effect is to make you sleepy but arousable, able to breathe on your own, and not keenly aware of your surroundings. With MAC, you'll have only a cloudy memory of what happened during the procedure. The effects don't linger in your body, so you can be talking and moving around within minutes—an hour at the most.

All patients have different dosage requirements before they enter twilight sleep. Under sedation, you'll be relaxed but not completely unconscious. Sometimes the difference between the two states is not quite clear, and people react differently to sedation. The same dose of drug, for instance, may produce sedation in one patient but loss of consciousness in another. Careful, customized dosing to achieve the perfect balance is the expertise of the anesthesia provider.

 The amount, or dosage, of sedative medication depends on the patient's
- *Body size*
- *Existing medical conditions, such as obesity, sleep apnea, and drug or alcohol habits*
- *Anxiety level*
- *Surgical requirement*

Sedated patients may fall in and out of sleep during surgery. If you become increasingly aware of your surroundings, you'll be given more sedation. You should not feel any pain, because the surgeon and anesthesiologist are careful to keep you calm and pain-free. If you do experience pain while under MAC, you can speak up so that more local anesthetic can be applied.

Halves and Parts: Regional Anesthesia

Regional anesthesia is the placement of an anesthetic medication to block sensation or movement in the part of the body undergoing surgery. This type of anesthesia is preferred to general anesthesia—in which patients become completely unconscious—in procedures *where there is a choice*. Regional anesthesia has a valuable place in many operations and is used with patients who may have some special risk associated with general anesthesia.

Regional anesthesia mainly involves applying a local anesthetic around nerves. In this case the local anesthetic "bathes" the nerves coming out of the spinal cord or the large nerves that control your arms and legs. The local anesthetic blocks the pain signals and, depending on the dosage, can block movement. The amount of anesthesia can be adjusted not only for the duration of the surgery but also for pain management after surgery.

There are three types of regional anesthesia: **spinal, epidural,** and **peripheral nerve blocks.** We'll look at all three next.

The Security Blanket for the Brain

Thin layers of membrane (tissue) called **meninges** surround the brain and the spinal cord. These three layers—the pia, arachnoid, and dura—blanket the brain and spinal cord. The **subarachnoid space** is the space between the arachnoid and the pia. It is filled with **cerebrospinal fluid** (CSF), which cushions the brain and spinal cord from sudden shocks and movements. The space above the dura is called the epidural space. (The Latin prefix *epi-* means "above." *Epidural* means "above the dura.")

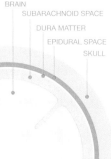

BRAIN
SUBARACHNOID SPACE
DURA MATTER
EPIDURAL SPACE
SKULL

From the Waist Down

Spinal and epidural anesthetics can block pain or movement in the lower body. They are popular for procedures performed at the waist and below. For example, hernia repair or hip surgery can be done with a spinal or epidural.

The most frequent use of spinals and epidurals is in obstetrics. Women in labor can rest comfortably with an epidural while they focus on the birthing process, rather than on the pain. If a cesarean section is required, a strong dose of local anesthetic is needed to increase the intensity of the pain block. (Read more about it in chapter 10.)

No Germs, Please—We're Operating

Every surgery is a **sterile** procedure. This means *no germs* are allowed anywhere near the patient. Before entering the operating room, surgeons and nurses remove their street clothes and put on scrub suits, masks, caps, and shoe covers. Next they vigorously wash their hands and arms up to the elbows, using a special **bacteria**-killing solution. Then they don gowns and gloves. Except for the scrubs, all these items of clothing are disposable. The gowns and gloves are individually pre-packaged and worn immediately before approaching a patient. This means that surgeons and nurses can't touch anything outside the "sterile field"—a demarcated area immediately around a patient. Any person in the room not properly gowned and gloved cannot go near the patient. Anesthesiologists wear **scrubs**, cap, and mask but not a sterile gown or gloves. Since they are not part of the "sterile field," anesthesiologists have to maintain a safe distance away from the site of surgery and not touch anything that is used on the patient.

Instruments used on the patient have to remain sterile throughout the procedure. Drapes and coverings surrounding the patient are also sterile. Today, many surgical instruments and all drapes used on the patient are disposable. Immediately after use, any device (such as a colonoscope, drill, or metal stabilizer for broken bones) or instruments to be reused are rinsed and soaked in a specially formulated detergent that kills bacteria. All metal instruments are placed in a high-temperature (49°C or 120°F), high-pressure steam-cleaning machine called an autoclave.

Position, Prep, and Placement

The process of placing spinal and epidural anesthetics requires patient cooperation—because it's all about position, position, position! Placement of the anesthetic can be done with you either sitting or lying on your side. The anesthesiologist will ask you to put yourself into a "slouch," "bad posture," or "cooked shrimp" position. These positions spread out the bones of your back (the **vertebrae**) so that the spinal or epidural needle can be neatly inserted in the small spaces between them.

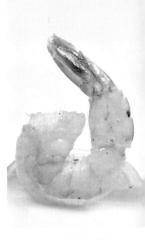

CURL YOUR BODY LIKE A COOKED SHRIMP.

(An autoclave is akin to a giant pressure cooker.) Delicate devices (colonoscope) are placed in an automatic cleaning machine. This sequential process kills not only bacteria but also the HIV and hepatitis viruses.

Maintaining sterility is an important protocol in every operating room. Sterile practice prevents infection and ensures the patient's safe recovery. Something as seemingly minor as an unmasked sneeze or cough can spread germs onto a surgical site.

A breach in sterility either in preparing instruments for surgery or during the procedure can have dire consequences for a patient. On rare occasions, an infection at the site of surgery can occur despite all precautions. The exact cause of infection is often hard to trace.

Early detection of an infection is essential because an infection can prevent a wound from healing and cause pain, redness, and soreness—or, worse yet, pus can build up in the operated area. If infection develops, the patient must take antibiotics for a few weeks. A non-healing wound may warrant a second operation to reopen the area and clean it out. If an infection is not controlled early on, it can spread throughout the body, resulting in **sepsis**. Sepsis means the bacteria has spread through the bloodstream into other organs like the kidneys, liver, lungs, heart, and brain. This is a serious condition that has to be aggressively treated with multiple antibiotics and long-term hospitalization. The worst consequence of uncontrolled sepsis is death.

Now you can understand why health-care practitioners cannot wear street clothes or shoes in an operating room!

Placement is done under sterile (super-clean) conditions. Your back is cleansed with a solution that kills germs on the skin. A sterile plastic drape, with a small opening to isolate the area for the procedure, is attached to the back. Then a pinch of local anesthetic numbs the skin site before the actual spinal or epidural needle is inserted.

Spinal

A spinal anesthetic is placed with a long, fine, hollow needle gently inserted into the lower back, below the level at which the spinal cord ends. A small amount of spinal fluid that is drawn out shows that the correct spot for insertion has been found. A local anesthetic is then injected into the space through the needle. A spinal is a one-time-only insertion, because the needle is removed after the local anesthetic is delivered.

Epidural

Epidural needles are slightly larger than those used in spinals. A syringe with some air is attached to the epidural needle. The epidural needle and the air-filled syringe are advanced together ever so slightly—millimeter by millimeter. When the air-filled syringe easily collapses, it indicates that the epidural space has been located. A fine, pliable plastic

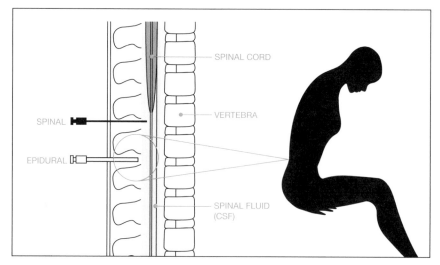

WHERE THE NEEDLES GO

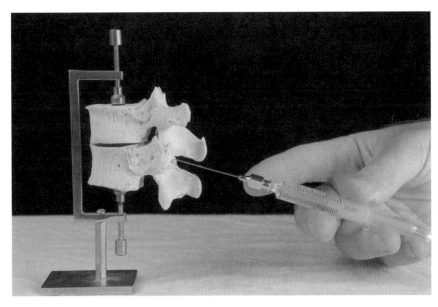

A PRECISE SPOT HAS TO BE LOCATED.

catheter is then threaded through the needle, and the needle is removed over the catheter. Only 4 to 6 centimeters (1 to 2 inches) of the catheter remain in the epidural space. The epidural catheter is then taped to the back and hangs over your shoulder.

The epidural catheter looks like a piece of angel hair pasta sticking out of your back. It is so unnoticeable that you can lie on your back comfortably.

The anesthesiologist can inject local anesthetic through the catheter repeatedly, or she can attach it to a pump for a continuous flow of anesthetic. An epidural also differs from a spinal because it can be placed in the upper or lower back, and it can be combined with a general anesthetic so that the patient receives less general anesthetic. Removing the catheter is easy; the anesthesia provider simply gives it a tug, and out it comes.

Combined Spinal and Epidural Technique

The combined spinal-epidural is a unique anesthetic technique. A spinal needle is placed through the larger epidural needle. A dose of

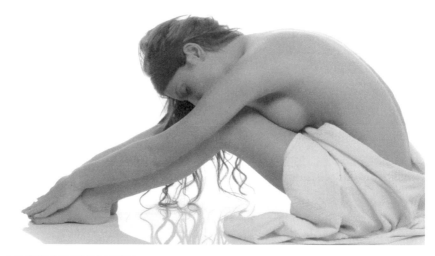

A FLEXIBLE BACK IS A BONUS.

medication is given through the spinal needle, and then the epidural catheter is threaded through. The benefit is the rapid onset of a nerve block from a spinal, combined with the repeated dosing through the epidural catheter.

⚠ *Keep in mind that these tried-and-true techniques have been performed on millions of people. The thought of a needle in the back often scares patients, though. That's understandable, but in the right circumstances the benefits of a regional anesthetic outweigh the risks. Remember that the site of needle insertion is numbed heavily, and sedation is commonly given before the procedure begins. The sedative medication causes* **amnesia,** *so most patients don't remember the details. (Women in labor are not given sedation, to protect the baby. Sedation is also withheld during a C-section prior to delivery of the baby.) Regaining your wits promptly after surgery and lasting pain control are good reasons for choosing a regional anesthetic.*

It's unlikely that you'll actually see any of the surgical procedure, because a drape will be placed in front of you, blocking your view. You'll also be given twilight sleep sedation to make you less anxious.

NOT FOR EVERYONE

Let's touch on some of the reasons a spinal or epidural wouldn't be used:

1. You simply refuse to have one.
2. You have anatomical problems in the back (spina bifida, Harrington rods, severe scoliosis).
3. You have a bleeding disorder (hemophilia, von Willebrand disease).
4. You take a medication that interferes with blood clotting, such as heparin, clopidogrel (Plavix), or warfarin (Coumadin).
5. You suffer from specific heart problems that make receiving epidurals and spinals more risky (severe aortic stenosis, idiopathic hypertrophic cardiomyopathy).
6. There is a localized infection at the skin site on your back.
7. You have an untreated blood infection.
8. You have signs of severe **dehydration**, bleeding, or unstable blood pressure.

A UNIQUE HEADACHE

A **spinal headache** is the most common complication that can result from a spinal or epidural needle placement. Young women are more prone to this than older patients. The cause of the headache is a leakage of cerebrospinal fluid (CSF) through a hole in the dura. Epidural needles are large, and the epidural space is about 6 millimeters (0.24 inch) wide. If the anesthesiologist inadvertently advances the needle beyond the epidural space, and makes a hole in the dura, a CSF leak occurs. This is called a "wet tap," or **dural puncture**.

The most common symptom is a "positional" headache—one that gets worse with sitting up and improves with lying down. Fortunately, the situation is easy to treat with bed rest and pain medicines, and by drinking lots of water and caffeinated beverages. At times it stops spontaneously within a few days.

A faster treatment, though, is the **epidural blood patch**. Blood is taken under sterile conditions from an arm vein and injected through an epidural needle placed above the leak site. The blood clots over the hole in the dura and patches up the CSF leak. The headache is relieved within minutes in more than 80 percent of patients.

WHAT? A NEEDLE IN THE BACK?!

Patients tend to worry when it comes to needles and often ask the anesthesiologist, "Am I going to be paralyzed?" The fear comes from the idea that a needle is going right into your spinal cord. The needle, when put in correctly, does not touch the spinal cord.

⚠️ *Complications are incredibly rare. A spinal cord injury may result from bleeding in the epidural space, resulting in a hematoma—a localized blood clot. Unless the patient has a bleeding problem or is on a blood thinner (Coumadin, heparin), there's less than a one in one million chance of this happening. Infection or epidural abscess (a localized collection of bacteria and pus) is reported to occur in one in ten thousand placements—more likely in patients left with catheters for several days or in those with immune system problems. These are emergency situations that require prompt recognition and the intervention of a neurosurgeon.*

What If the Block Is Not 100 Percent?

Sometimes spinal or epidural anesthesia leaves patchy areas of the body unblocked because of uneven distribution of the local anesthetic. This may also happen with a peripheral nerve block. (See the next section.)

The anesthesiologist and surgeon always test the anesthesia before starting. The block may be redone or general anesthesia can always be given, so under no circumstance will you feel the surgery.

Just an Arm or a Leg: Peripheral Nerve Block

Peripheral nerve blocks are an increasingly popular form of anesthesia. A nerve block involves placement of a local anesthetic around the nerves that supply the surgical site. The numbing from the block can also continue to relieve pain after surgery. Sometimes catheters can be placed near nerves for a continuous supply of local anesthetic through a pump. For orthopedic surgery, nerve blocks are an excellent way to receive anesthesia.

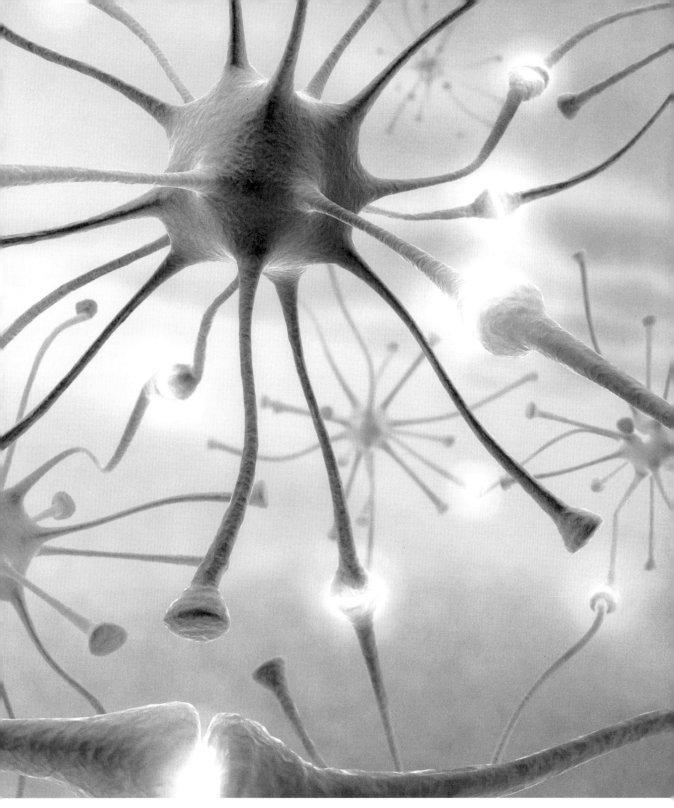

A NETWORK OF NERVES

Anesthesiologists have a complete knowledge of the anatomy of the nerves throughout the body. Proper placement of regional anesthesia takes time and expertise. An anesthesiologist does this by using anatomical landmarks on the surface of the body. The nerves that need to be blocked can be precisely located with an ultrasound probe or a nerve stimulator device.

An ultrasound probe allows the anesthesiologist to see the target nerves on a monitor screen while a needle is advanced. When the point of the needle is seen to be closest to the target nerves, a dose of local anesthetic is injected through the needle. The ultrasound technique allows precise placement of local anesthetic for a good-quality block.

The nerve stimulator is a device that sends out a small, low-voltage electric current from the tip of a needle. As the needle moves closer to the desired nerve, it stimulates the nerve. The muscles supplied by the nerve begin to twitch. The local anesthetic is injected into the spot where the most twitching with the lowest amount of electrical current is seen.

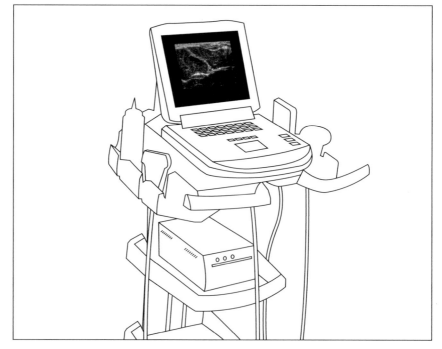

AN ULTRASOUND MACHINE

After placement of a nerve block is complete, your arm or leg will start to feel warm and heavy. A feeling of dissociation from your limb begins to take place—you may feel like your leg or arm is not yours. As the block wears off after surgery, you will regain the ability to sense and move your limb within a few hours.

⚠ *As with any form of regional anesthesia, there is a possibility of **block failure**, infection, bleeding, nerve injury, or **toxicity** from large doses of local anesthetic. The decision to use regional anesthesia depends on whether the benefits outweigh the risks for you as an individual.*

Totally Out: General Anesthesia

Most people's ideas about anesthesia come from TV shows and movies: a patient is shown lying on an operating table, completely "out." The anesthesiologist is sitting quietly behind surgical drapes, and all the focus is on the surgeon. That's what general anesthesia looks like to the observer.

But by breaking the process down to its parts, you'll see that it's more complex. The basic components of general anesthesia are:

- **Hypnosis:** loss of consciousness
- **Analgesia:** absence of pain
- **Amnesia:** absence of memory
- **Muscle relaxation:** absence of movement

The first three components are absolutely essential for a successful general anesthetic. General anesthesia is a "cocktail" of anesthetic gas, narcotics, memory blockers, **hypnotics** (medications that cause sleep), and muscle relaxants—each carefully dosed to the individual patient. Anesthetic gases block chemical transmissions in the brain and spinal cord. The gases can decrease consciousness, inhibit memory and pain, and stop movement. The other drugs mentioned compound the effect of the gases.

The Process

The general anesthetic process can be divided into three components: In adults, giving anesthetic medications through an **intravenous line**, or IV, is the usual method of **induction**, or starting the process. First an IV is inserted, then a mask is placed over the nose and mouth. You are

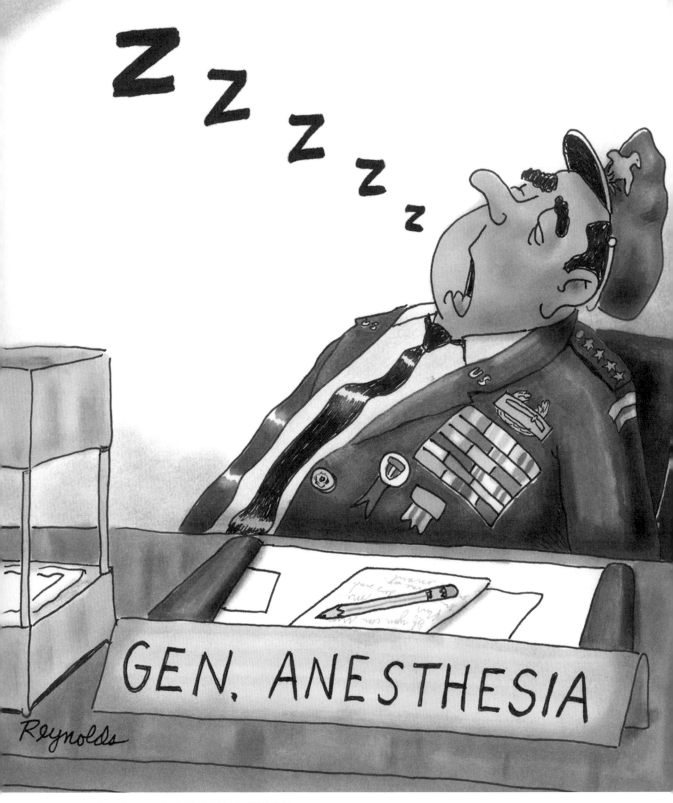

GENERAL ANESTHESIA IS COMPLETELY OUT!

asked to take deep breaths. This process fills your lungs with 100 per-cent oxygen. It takes less than half a minute for a patient to become un-conscious from IV medications, because they are placed directly into the bloodstream and travel right to the brain.

It is often hard to place an IV line in a fully awake child, so general anesthesia in young children is started by having them first inhale gases through a mask. (See chapter 11.) Once the young patient is unconscious from the gas, the IV placement can be done without any distress.

Maintenance of general anesthesia is achieved with a combination of IV medications and inhaled gases carefully measured for each pa-tient's needs.

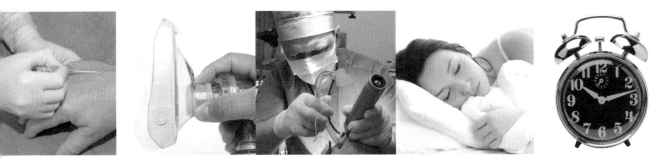

Emergence means waking up from general anesthesia. The deliv-ery of gases and medicines are stopped and allowed to exit the body through the lungs, kidneys, and liver. You gradually wake up from your sleep in the operating room or recovery room.

Each major part of the general anesthetic process—induction, main-tenance, and emergence—is a critical time that requires expertise and attention. Your anesthesiologist will be there to make sure that all goes well.

Breathe Easy: Airway Management

One of the most important skills of an anesthesiologist is **airway man-agement**. This term broadly includes all the maneuvers and devices used to maintain and ensure unobstructed movement of oxygen in and carbon dioxide out of the body. This is called **ventilation**, and it's critical to life.

Anesthetic gases and medications slow breathing, and at certain doses they can even stop breathing altogether. If a patient is deprived of oxygen, it can lead to brain damage and cardiac arrest within minutes. It is the responsibility of the anesthesiologist to optimize blood oxygen levels and keep air passages unobstructed. Anesthesiologists have all sorts of equipment for this purpose.

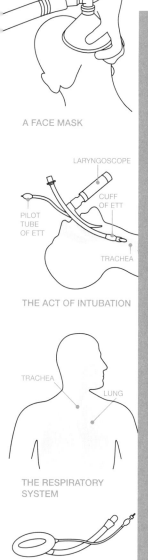

A FACE MASK

LARYNGOSCOPE

CUFF OF ETT

PILOT TUBE OF ETT

TRACHEA

THE ACT OF INTUBATION

TRACHEA

LUNG

THE RESPIRATORY SYSTEM

A LARYNGEAL MASK AIRWAY

Breathing Passages

The airway includes the mouth, structures in the mouth (teeth and tongue), and the larynx (voice box) down to the trachea (windpipe). Normally, our vocal cords close to protect us from having solids and liquids enter our trachea. When solids or liquids enter the trachea—"go down the wrong way"—we cough or, worse, choke.

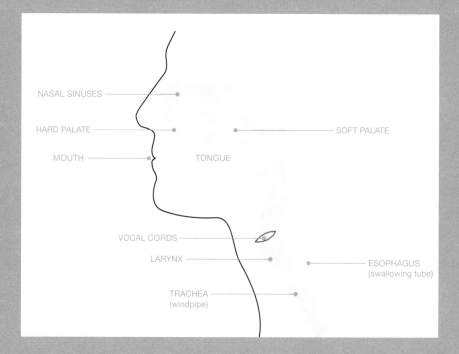

NASAL SINUSES

HARD PALATE

MOUTH

TONGUE

SOFT PALATE

VOCAL CORDS

LARYNX

ESOPHAGUS (swallowing tube)

TRACHEA (windpipe)

To protect the airway, a rigid, clear, plastic **face mask** can be placed over the patient's mouth and nose, a tube with an inflatable cuff at the end (laryngeal mask airway, or LMA) can be placed to sit snugly over the larynx, or a breathing tube (**endotracheal tube**, or ETT) can be inserted directly into the trachea. A source of oxygen (anesthesia machine) is always connected to the face mask, LMA, or endotracheal tube.

The placement of an endotracheal tube into the trachea is called **intubation**. Anesthesiologists are trained to place the tubes easily and efficiently. They are experts at this, and they use a variety of devices—laryngoscope, fiberoptic scope, GlideScope, or Airtraq—to do this.

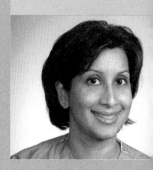

PanchLines

Dr. Dhar Explains: Overcoming the Challenge

If you are told that you are a "difficult intubation" before or after a general anesthetic, be absolutely sure to mention it to any surgeons and anesthesiologists treating you in the future. This will ensure that they take proper precautions before beginning your anesthesia. Difficulty may stem from obesity or anatomic features.

Fancy new devices are on the market today that have increased the safety of intubation. That means there is less chance of dental injury, missed tube insertion, or sore throat for you.

Anybody who is a professional singer needs to alert the anesthesiologist. Extra care of the vocal cords is a must. Discuss with your doctor if intubation can be avoided altogether or if another technique can be used.

If you experience **sleep apnea** and use a home breathing device, it is a good idea to bring your machine along or at least know your settings so that your sleep apnea can be addressed during aftercare.

The circumstances in which a person is brought to the operating room also matter a great deal. Emergency surgery can be riskier than a planned procedure. For example, brain surgery that takes place shortly after a blood vessel ruptures is far riskier than a planned procedure to clip off the same weak vessel before it bursts.

Emergencies are exactly what they are—emergencies. But when a surgery or other procedure is planned, you want to make sure you get in the best possible medical condition ahead of time. This is a good time to quit smoking, as it will clear up your lungs. Be sure to take your medications to control high blood pressure, asthma, or diabetes in the time before the procedure. You'll also want to discuss your general health and lifestyle habits with your doctor well in advance of surgery.

Rx Prescriptives: Be a Better Consumer

☐ **What type of anesthesia is commonly provided for the procedure you are having? Ask your doctor.** _____

_____

☐ **What type of anesthesia is planned for you? (It may be different from what is routine.)** _____

_____

☐ **What are your concerns or fears about the type of anesthesia planned for you? Discuss this with your doctor.** _____

_____

☐ **What type of anesthesia would you prefer to have? A general, regional, or sedation? Discuss the options with your doctor.** _____

_____

☐ **Think about any issues you had with a previous type of anesthetic that you want to avoid in the future (e.g., difficult intubation, difficult spinal placement, claustrophobia with face mask placement, sore throat).** _____

_____

it's showtime! { what
to expect

CHAPTERTHREE

the countdown:
diving in

The decision has been made: you're going to
have surgery. Whether it has been planned for weeks
or you just learned that the procedure must take place
tomorrow, you will certainly have met your surgeon. But
you might have no idea who will handle your anesthesia.

Don't worry! The anesthesiologist is as well prepared
as your surgeon. Even with just a few minutes before
emergency surgery, you and your loved ones can ask
questions to better understand your anesthetic. Your
range of anesthetic options will be explained so you can
accept with confidence what lies ahead.

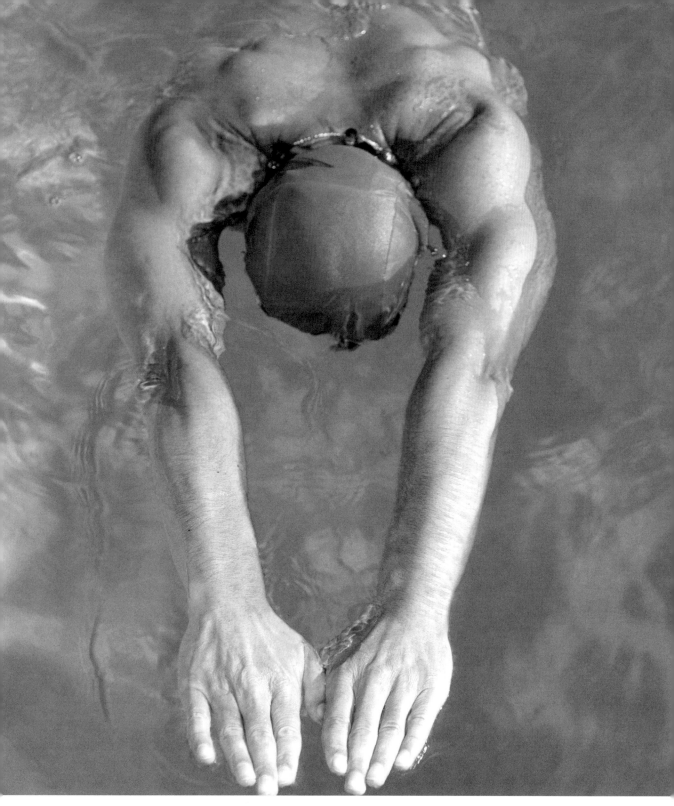

HEAD FOR THE FINISH LINE.

YOUR COMPLETE MEDICAL HISTORY HELPS PLAN FUTURE CARE.

First Things First: Doctors Learn about You

First, your overall physical condition must be assessed. This process begins two to three weeks before a scheduled surgery or other procedure. There are several steps in this pre-operative evaluation, depending on your overall health and the type of procedure planned.

Otherwise healthy patients with no evidence of disease based on their history or physical exam do not need a battery of medical tests. People with co-existing medical problems (such as heart disease or diabetes) and those patients facing risky or extensive surgery require further medical work-up.

Let's say you're scheduled for hip replacement next month. The surgeon and anesthesia provider must first learn about any health issues you have. You'll be asked to fill out an extensive questionnaire about your past medical history, family health history, current physical limitations, exercise habits, tobacco and alcohol use, specific body systems (heart, lungs, stomach, brain, kidneys, joints), medication, allergies, previous surgeries, and so on. The questionnaire may be a form that you fill out in a doctor's office, it may be conducted as a telephone interview, or it may be something you complete online. It's important to be honest. Once you have completed the questionnaire you'll receive information that explains how to prepare for the surgery, including fasting and medication instructions. Some hospitals direct you to their Web sites for further explanations.

Some people visit the hospital pre-surgical testing center to give blood and/or urine samples for laboratory tests, or to get a chest X-ray or an **electrocardiogram** (EKG). Specialized blood tests and exams may be done, depending on your age, general health status, and the type of procedure you're having.

⚠ *Follow your paper trail. Whether pre-surgical tests are done in the hospital or elsewhere, it is important to make sure the results have been forwarded to your doctors. In our increasingly complex health-care world, it is not unusual for tests and medical records to be mislaid— especially when multiple medical facilities and insurance providers are involved. Call the clinic or lab to verify that all test results and other records have been sent to your surgical team.*

Another good way to be your own medical advocate is to acquire a full set of your medical records and test results, and keep them up to date. Carry them with you every time you visit a health-care provider.

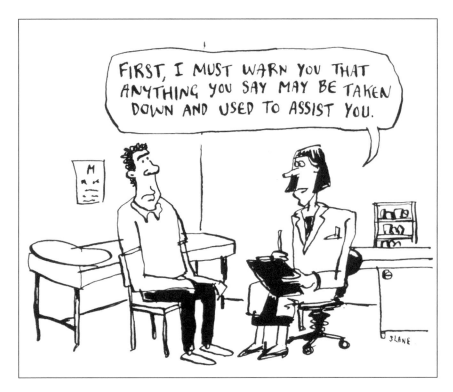

Clearing the Way

Some patients must obtain a **medical clearance** note before surgery can be performed. This important document provides a recent evaluation by a specialist or by your primary care physician. It includes suggestions for medical management during your surgery. It also highlights your most pertinent medical problems and health conditions. For example, if you're at risk of heart disease, you may be asked to see a cardiologist for further evaluation. A medical clearance includes interpretation of a cardiac stress test, echocardiogram, cardiac catheterization, EKG, pulmonary function tests, chest X-ray, and appropriate blood tests.

Mixing Anesthesia with Viagra, Levetra, or Cialis

Medications such as Viagra (sildenefil), Levitra (vardenafil), and Cialis (tadalafil) work by opening up blood vessels and increasing blood flow.

You must tell the anesthesiologist if you have recently taken any of these medications. Anesthesiologists sometimes use medications called nitrates (nitroglycerin and nitroprusside) to control a patient's blood pressure during an operation. A drug interaction between nitrates and these popular erectile dysfunction (ED) drugs can cause a patient's blood pressure to become dangerously low.

It is best to discontinue use of these drugs at least twenty-four hours before surgery to avoid interaction with other blood pressure medications.

Learn What Lies Ahead

If the surgeon has any additional concerns about your health, you may be required to meet an anesthesia provider before the date of surgery. (Of course, you're always welcome to request a visit with the anesthesiologist!) The person you meet may be the anesthesiologist who will manage your surgery or another person on the A (anesthesia) Team.

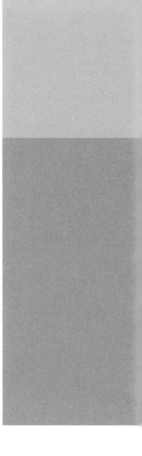

Anesthesia providers consider the pre-operative period a critical time. They want to learn all they can about you so they can improve or maintain your health before surgery, as well as prepare the anesthesia plan. The pre-anesthesia visit has several goals:

- Assess the status of your health.
- Assess any special anesthetic risks that you may have, such as a difficult airway.
- Ensure your readiness for anesthesia. This includes both your physical and psychological status.
- Devise a mutually agreeable anesthesia plan with you, your loved ones, and the anesthesia team.
- Reduce your anxiety about anesthesia.
- Discuss the various anesthetic options available for your particular type of surgery or procedure.

All your health information, test results, and laboratory data are collected in a **chart** and given to the anesthesiologist assigned to you on the day of surgery. In some hospitals or centers, an anesthesia consent form must be signed. In other places, the anesthetic consent is understood to be part of the **surgical consent form**. Keep in mind that in emergency situations, your health-care proxy or family members may provide consent. A consent form is an acknowledgment that you understand the procedure, the alternative options, as well as the risks and benefits of an intervention.

Before the surgery, talk with your surgeon about the anesthetic specialists who are available to you. This is particularly important if you have medical problems in addition to the one for which you are being treated. In most hospitals, certain anesthesiologists work regularly with certain surgeons. Working with the same colleagues over time establishes an understanding of each other's expectations and style, and that bond makes for a flawless routine.

 Ask your surgeon which anesthesiologists regularly work with her, or who is most proficient with the anesthesia for your type of surgery. The surgeon can arrange for a particular anesthesiologist with the expertise necessary for your care.

Fasting Guidelines: Food, Drink, and Medications

The anesthesiologist will insist that you not eat or drink anything based on **nil per os** (NPO) guidelines. These guidelines tell you how long you have to abstain from foods and liquids before surgery.

 *It is critical that you strictly follow the NPO guidelines. The most important reason for keeping your stomach empty is so you won't aspirate (inhale) vomited food into your lungs. **Aspiration** can cause serious damage to your lungs and may lead to death. The anesthetic drugs reduce your natural inclination to protect your airway, because you are not fully aware or totally conscious that you have vomited. Be sure to tell your anesthesiologist if you have **gastroesophogeal reflux disease** (GERD).*

Fried or fatty foods or meat take a long time to digest. That's why a fasting period of at least eight hours before surgery is required after such a meal. A light meal consists of dry toast and clear liquid. Milk is like solid food, because it takes time to be digested and leave the stomach. No alcohol is allowed before surgery, as it worsens dehydration.

Continue your regular medications unless you are told otherwise. Diabetics are given special instructions about insulin dosing and oral agents on the morning of surgery. Be sure to discuss this matter with your

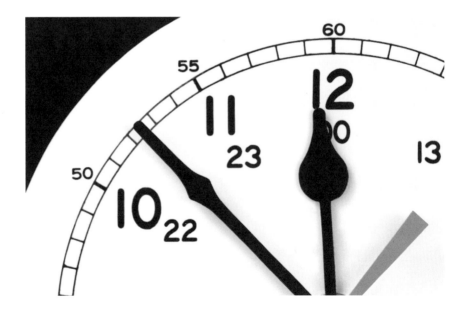

surgeon or anesthesiologist before the surgery. That way you can be sure that you take only what is appropriate on the day of the procedure. Typically, however, if you must take your medication before surgery, it is fine to take it with small sips of water.

Dr. Dhar Advises: Morning, Noon, or Night?

The later in the day your surgery is scheduled, the more dehydrated you will become. That's because you can't drink fluids after a certain point. The earlier in the day that a same-day (or ambulatory) procedure is done, the more likely you are to return home by dark to recover. Sometimes your request for an early procedure cannot be accommodated because of patient volume and other surgical priorities, but it never hurts to ask. You should inquire about receiving intravenous hydration if you are required to wait a long time for your procedure.

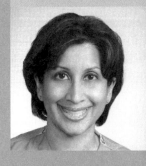

General Fasting Guidelines before a Procedure

Item	Period of Time to Fast after Consumption
Clear liquids (water, fruit juices without pulp, carbonated beverages, clear tea, black coffee)	2 hours
Breast milk	4 hours
Infant formula	6 hours (4 hours if under 6 months old)
Cow milk	6 hours (4 hours if under 6 months old)
Non-clear liquid (coffee with milk)	6 hours
Light meal (dry toast and clear liquid)	6 hours
Solid food	8 hours

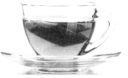

All this preparation is for *your* big moment. You are going to be the center of attention on that day. Your thoughts, concerns, fears, and hopes have all been laid out. Each person taking care of you wants the best outcome no matter what you have to encounter. Every detail about you has been combed through. It is a special moment in your life because you have put in so much time and effort to prepare. You have talked to your doctors, read about the surgery, followed instructions, and gone through tests—now it's time to take a deep breath as the moment approaches. Yes, you *can* make it a positive experience. The most important goal is for you to come out better and stronger. You can then look back satisfied that you did your best.

Your anesthesiologist is a person whom you will meet yet may not remember because of the brevity of the encounter. But for that doctor, at that particular moment, you are the star. This doctor has to learn everything she can about you thoroughly and expeditiously. It is unlike an encounter with doctors who may have known you for days, months, or years. The care the anesthesia providers give is brief, but intense.

Ironically, if you can't recall details about the anesthesia, the doctor has done a good job.

(Rx) **Prescriptives:** Be a Better Consumer

☐ **Write down a timeline with all your medical history.** _____

_____

☐ **Make a list of all your current health problems.** _____

_____

☐ **Make a list of all the medications you take. This includes herbal supplements.**

_____

_____

☐ **Do you need or want to meet with an anesthesiologist before your scheduled procedure?** _____

_____

☐ **Does the anesthesia provider have all your pertinent medical test results before your procedure day?** _____

_____

☐ **Are you clear about when you are supposed to stop eating before a procedure?**

_____

_____

Your Planning Calendar
Use this to schedule tests and doctor visits before surgery.

SUNDAY	MONDAY	TUESDAY	WEDNESDAY	THURSDAY	FRIDAY	SATURDAY

CHAPTER FOUR

clean
and serene:
the operating
room

A wave of emotions might sweep over you when you enter an **operating room** (OR) for the first time—the place where your surgery will take place. Often, the room is not what you imagined, or what you've seen in the movies or on TV. You might feel intimidated or downright scared. Some patients experience rapid heartbeat, break into a cold sweat, or shake uncontrollably.

On the other hand, you might feel relaxed, confident that you are in good hands, and looking forward to the results of a life-improving event. Knowing what to expect will help you to experience this more positive reaction.

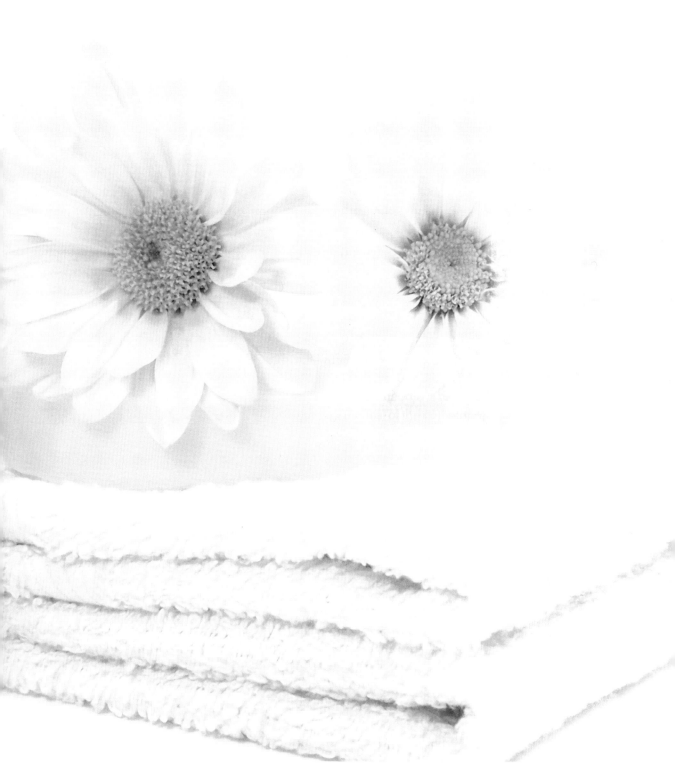

TAKE A DEEP BREATH AND RELAX.

The Setup

The typical operating room is a sterile area. There are no frills in most ORs—no pretty pictures on the wall, no cheery drapes and rugs. The floor and walls are tiled, so that they can easily be washed. Color schemes are soft blues, grays, or plain white. Stainless steel tables and stools are scattered about. For a particular surgery, additional equipment may be brought in, such as cameras, video monitors, fluoroscopic machines, X-ray machines, and heart/lung bypass machines. (We look at common OR equipment in chapter 5.) Above all, the operating room and everything inside it are spotlessly clean and sterile.

An operating room in a surgical center or off-site location such as a doctor's office has a similar setup. It may be more spa-like in appearance, but it will certainly be clean and sterile.

You might be surprised by the cold temperature in the OR. Although you will remain warm under blankets and other covers, the cold air is maintained for the comfort of the people who work there for hours on end under uncomfortably hot, bright lights.

Who Are All These People?!

The essential personnel in the operating room are the surgeons, anesthesia providers, and nurses. Those helping the surgeon are surgical resident doctors or physician assistants. The A Team includes the senior anesthesiologist as well as a resident or certified registered nurse anesthetist (CRNA).

There may be other people standing about whom you don't recognize or understand why they are needed. Some may be medical students and representatives from medical instrument manufacturing companies. All these people can make the room seem crowded.

The nursing team in the OR is unique. Before a procedure, the nursing team prepares all the required instruments. A **scrub nurse** or a technician works alongside the surgeon to hand over instruments as they are needed. A **circulating nurse** moves about to help the surgeon, anesthesia provider, scrub nurse, and you, the patient. For example, the circulating nurse, or "circulator," makes sure that you're moved safely to and from the operating room; checks on the availability of specialized instruments

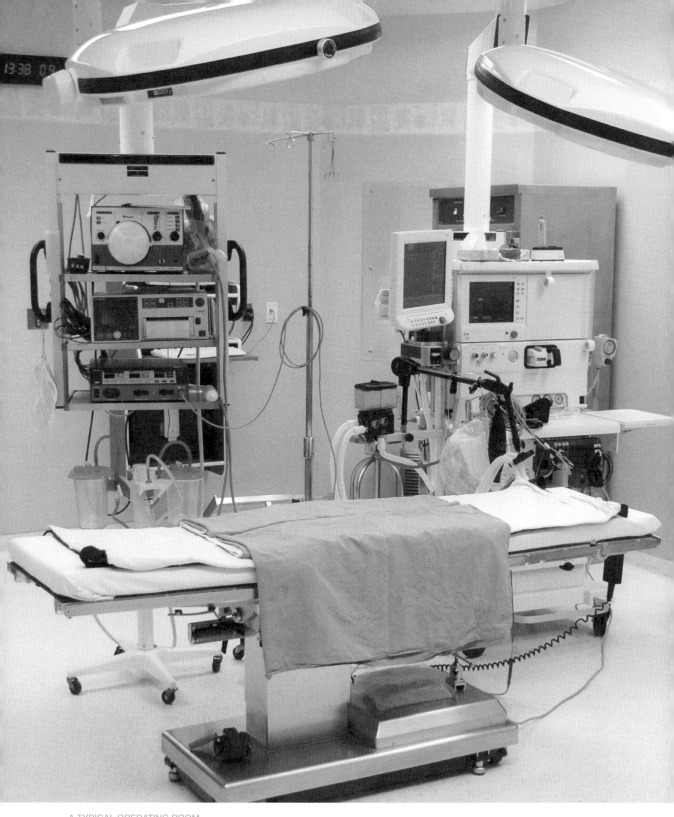

A TYPICAL OPERATING ROOM

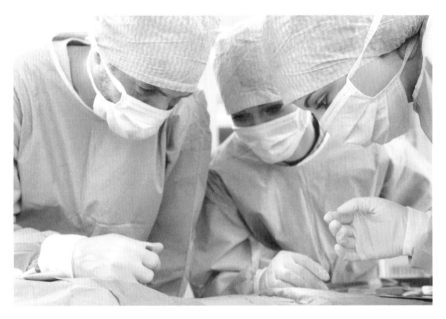

ALL EYES ARE ON YOU.

(orthopedic, gynecology, cardiac, and the like); operates diagnostic equipment such as cameras; and attends to the needs of the anesthesia provider, such as calling the blood bank if a transfusion is needed.

Together, the scrub nurse and the circulating nurse monitor the surgical and anesthesia teams to make sure that all instruments remain sterile during the procedure. At the end of a procedure, the nurses do an instrument count of the number of needles, clamps, and sponges used. After all, no one wants to leave a sponge or instrument inside the patient!

Everyone who works in an operating room is required to wear a lightweight outfit called scrubs. Over their scrubs, the surgeon and scrub nurse wear dense, sterile gowns. They may be standing directly under uncomfortably hot bright lights for hours on end, so the room is kept cold.

The only people who are not heavily gowned and gloved are the circulating nurse, the anesthesia provider, and you. The circulating nurse and anesthesiologist wear scrubs only. You, meanwhile, are in a hospital gown. Everyone working in the OR wears a mask over the mouth and nose, and a cap that covers the hair. All you can see of people's

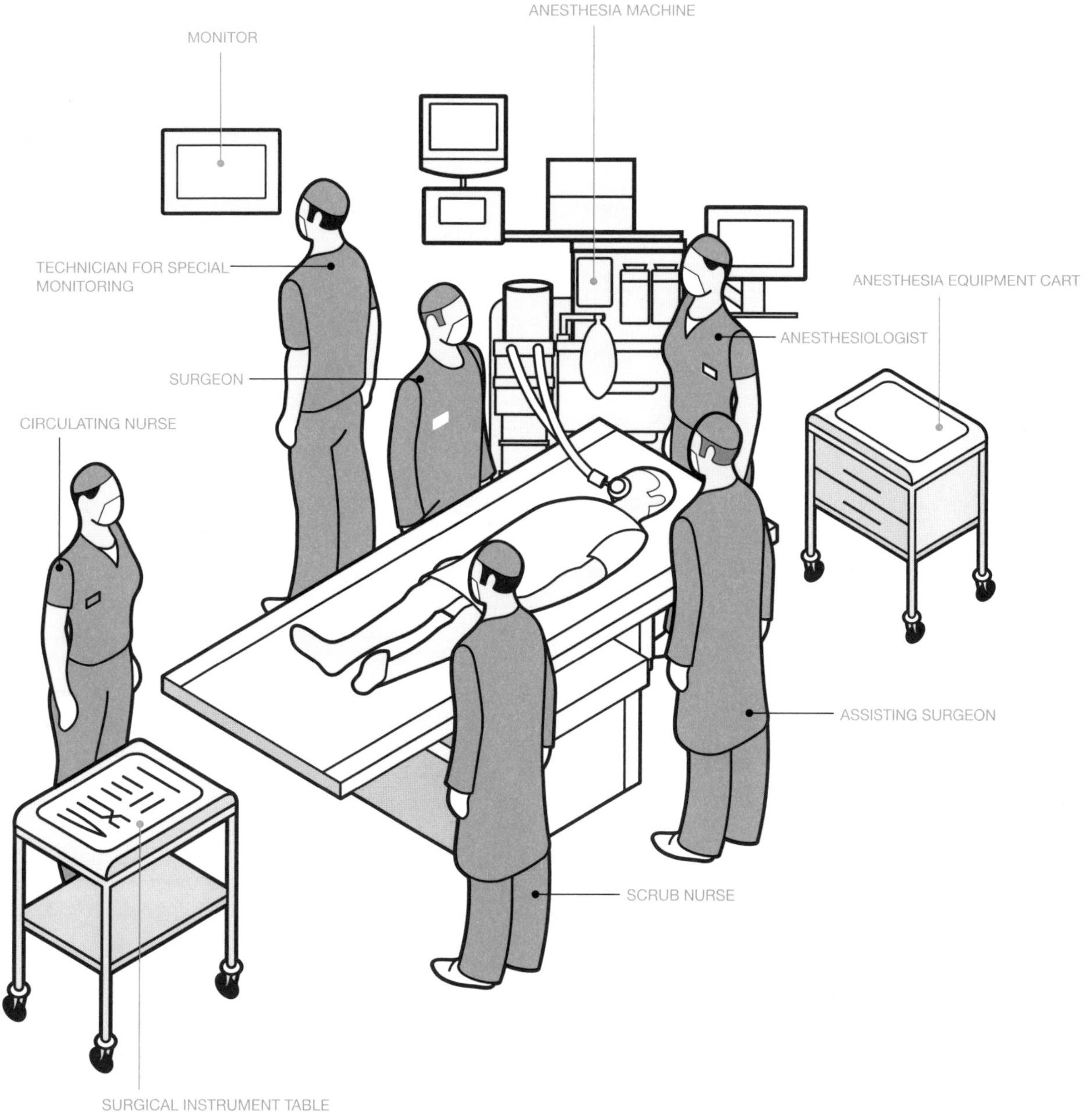

MONITOR

ANESTHESIA MACHINE

TECHNICIAN FOR SPECIAL
MONITORING

ANESTHESIA EQUIPMENT CART

ANESTHESIOLOGIST

SURGEON

CIRCULATING NURSE

ASSISTING SURGEON

SCRUB NURSE

SURGICAL INSTRUMENT TABLE

A VIEW OF ALL THE PEOPLE IN THE OPERATING ROOM

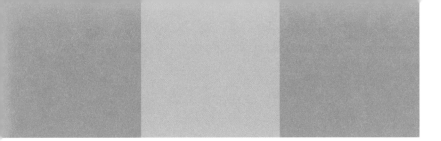

faces are their eyes. The cap and mask prevent germs or hair from traveling through the air. If someone sneezes or coughs, for example, the mask keeps airborne droplets from landing on the open surgical area.

Outside the OR: ID Check!

When you arrive outside the OR, the circulating nurse will ask you questions about your health that you probably have already answered many times during your surgical journey. Don't take offense or feel that you haven't been listened to before. This brief interview is conducted to make sure you are the correct patient, to confirm that you understand what type of procedure is to be done, to make sure the correct side of surgery is documented (for example, the right or left knee), to document that you have signed consent for the procedure, and to check again if you have any drug allergies or special requests. Everyone must be absolutely sure that you're the right patient for the right surgery.

 *A protocol called **time out** prevents wrong-patient/wrong-side surgery. Just before a procedure begins, all persons in the OR verify the patient's name, chart number, procedure, and exact site of surgery.*

If you're meeting the anesthesia provider for the first time in the OR, she will review the details of your medical chart and will ask about your current health status. Consider this interview as yet another measure of safety and reassurance.

This is also an opportunity to talk about your anesthesia preferences or concerns. There's no time like *now* to ask more questions or change your mind about a thing or two. You may have planned to have local anesthesia and sedation, but now, at the last minute, you may say, "I want a general anesthetic, please." The risks and benefits of another technique will be considered, and your wishes will be accommodated if possible. Anesthesiologists admire patients who choose to be active partners in the surgical process.

Dr. Dhar Notes: OR Deejays

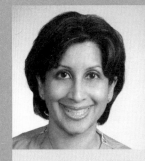

Many operating rooms today are equipped with sound systems to hook up iPods or play CDs, so don't be surprised if you hear music playing when you enter the operating room. It might be anything from classical to hip-hop to rock.

Anesthesiologists, surgeons, and nurses like to work with background music playing. Studies have shown that doctors work more efficiently with music.

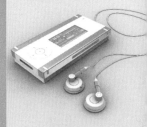

Anesthesiologists often act as OR deejays. Some anesthesiologists amass a large selection of music in their iPods or laptops just for this purpose. Surgeons may even prefer working with a particular anesthesiologist not only for her medical skill but also for her music choices.

Music relieves the tension in the room and lightens the atmosphere. It can be tailored to what's going on at the moment and who the patient is. When the patient is under general anesthesia, the genre can change depending on the stage of surgery—Mozart for opening, Armin van Buuren for closing.

But if things are not going well or get stressful, the music is a distraction and is turned off.

Crossing the Threshold

After you enter the OR, you are either transferred from the gurney that brought you or asked to lie on the operating table if you walked in. The first thing you notice is how narrow the table is. It's made this way so that the surgeon can easily reach both sides of your body. A snug strap is placed around you to make sure you don't fall off. Your arms may be extended outward on arm boards. This position makes it easier for the anesthesiologist to place on your body all the essential connections to monitors.

Some patients get anxious if they don't immediately see the surgeon in the operating room. Don't worry. Some surgeons like to enter the OR only when they are told that everything is ready for them to begin. In addition, surgeons know that anesthesiologists need time to place monitors, intravenous (IV) lines, nerve blocks, spinals, and epidurals after you arrive in the OR. Your surgeon may be out of the room to give the anesthesiologist the time and space to set up the equipment.

Rest assured that a member of the surgical team must always be present before anesthetic drugs are given. If your surgeon has not arrived in the OR when you enter, you may request that he be there for your reassurance before you are put to sleep.

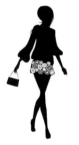

Compression Boots—Not for Walkin'

Boots may be placed around your calves before an operation. These boots intermittently inflate and compress your calves to prevent a blood clot (deep vein thrombus) from forming in your legs.

At this point, you may feel overwhelmed, exposed. It may seem like lots of people are touching you at the same time from all directions. Your arms are taken out of your hospital gown. Your upper body is exposed for a short time as cold, sticky EKG pads are applied to your skin. A **blood pressure cuff** is secured around your arm; the first time it tightens, you may feel uncomfortable. A lighted probe is placed on your fingertip to measure the oxygen level in your blood. Meanwhile, someone from the anesthesia team just placed a tight rubber tourniquet on your arm to find a vein in which to place an intravenous line. A sharp needle stick follows, and the tourniquet is released; the IV line is in. The needle stick is probably the most uncomfortable part of the process that you will remember before the anesthetic takes effect. *Note:* In some hospitals and surgery centers, the IV is placed by a nurse before you enter the OR.

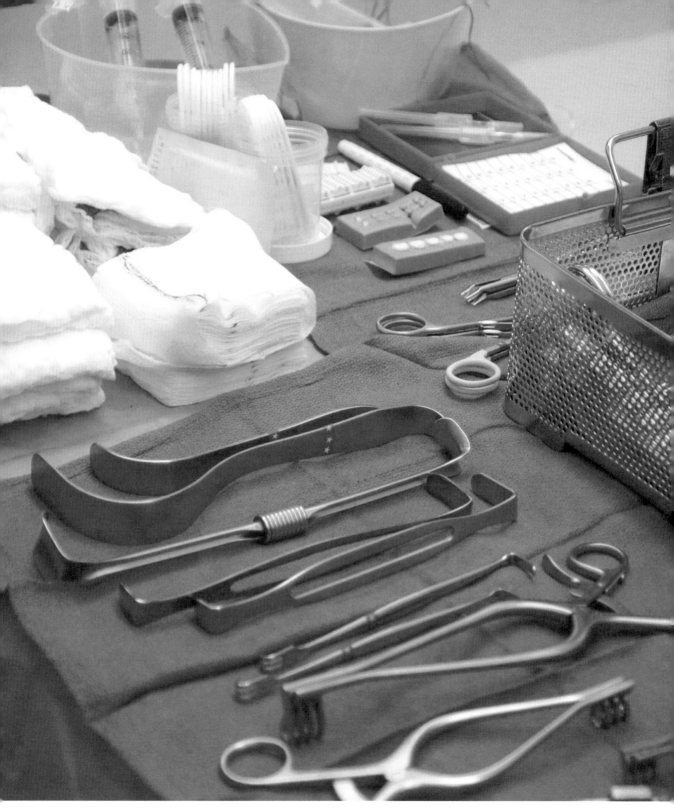

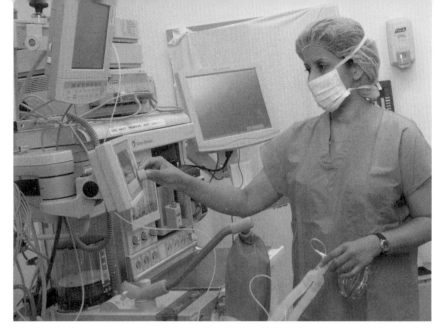

As all this activity swirls around you, you might be thinking about your future, your family, or simply getting through the moment. A staff member may have asked about something that you feel is very personal. Now some of your bodily functions are displayed on a monitor for everyone to see. It may be mind-boggling, and you may feel vulnerable. But have trust in the medical team: you are being well cared for.

Now you will receive the anesthesia and will enter into a different mental and physical world. Relax. A very special person—your anesthesiologist—is at the head of the operating table watching over you. You're safe.

Oftentimes a person's first encounter with an anesthesia provider and with anesthesia itself is very different from what he or she imagined it to be. The common depiction on television or the movies is an anesthesiologist sitting quietly behind drapes, with very little to say. Sometimes a one-liner like "the pressure is dropping" or "the oxygen level is dropping" is blurted out to the surgeon. And it seems like the TV surgeon is always the one frantically salvaging the patient from a crash. In reality, it is the anesthesiologist who brings the patient back from a nose dive—just as an airplane pilot regains control of an aircraft. The anesthesiologist is the doctor who can control the blood pressure and oxygen level, jump-start the heart, and give back blood when there is bleeding.

Perhaps someday the "hypospray" that Dr. McCoy used in *Star Trek* will be an anesthetic reality. It looked like a large pen and had no needle. On the television series, when Dr. McCoy pressed one of these gadgets on someone's neck, instantly the person felt relaxed, became unconscious, and felt no pain. Sounds like an anesthesia dream machine! An instrument like that would certainly make a lot of anesthetics used today obsolete. But until that happens, anesthesiologists will continue to handle your care.

Rx **Prescriptives:** Be a Better Consumer

☐ Ask if the operating room can be warmed up before you go in for your procedure. _____

_____

☐ Ask who each person in the procedure area is and what his or her role will be.

_____

☐ Make sure someone has verified what procedure you are having and what side you are having surgery on. _____

_____

☐ Ask if your music preference can be played to help you relax. _____

_____

☐ Ask to have the music volume turned down if that would help you relax. _____

_____

CHAPTERFIVE

watching over you:
monitors and measures

Human eyes and ears are needed to watch you—to monitor you—under anesthesia. Even watching your chest rise and fall with each breath is monitoring.

Human monitoring is a critical part of good anesthetic care. But technology extends the anesthesia provider's eyes and ears to keep track of what's happening inside the patient's body. Technology helps patients through complex surgeries; it also helps them to feel comfortable and safe. This is the role of medical **monitors**. With them, the anesthesiologist can not only keep track of what the surgeon is doing but also concentrate on things such as dosing medication.

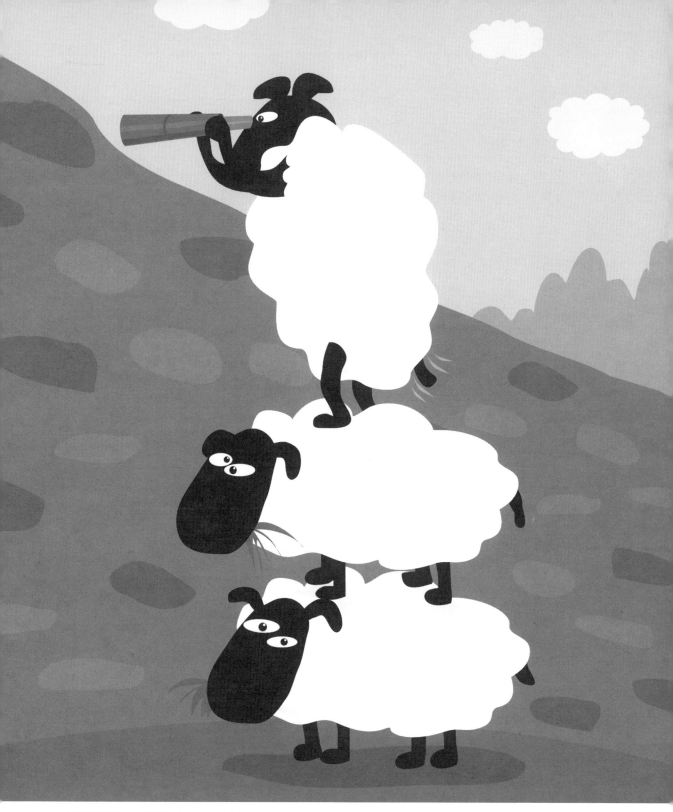

ANESTHESIA PROVIDERS ARE ALWAYS ON THE LOOKOUT.

The displays and sounds of monitors give information about what's going on inside the body during surgery. Since this is vital information, it is called vital signs. These include blood pressure, heart rate/rhythm, oxygen level, breathing rate, and body temperature. Vital signs respond to the effects of anesthesia and surgery, but the actions taken by the medical team have to be based on clinical judgment as well as numbers displayed. Different alarms help anesthesiologists respond promptly to changes that may not be apparent to the eye. For example, the **pulse oximeter** can detect a lowering of oxygen level long before a patient's skin turns blue. The level of monitoring is expanded depending on the patient's medical condition and the type of surgery.

Your Body Functions on Display

In the operating room, you'll be attached to what are known as **standard monitors**. These include an electrocardiograph, blood pressure cuff, pulse oximeter, capnograph, and temperature sensors. This section describes standard monitors and illustrates some of the ways in which anesthesiologists measure vital signs to ensure your safety.

Electrocardiograph: The Rhythm of the Heart

The electrocardiograph, or EKG, monitors your heart function. It measures your heart rate and rhythm. Adhesive pads with a conducting gel are attached to specific parts of your chest. The pads are connected to wires that transmit electrical signals detected from your heart and displayed on a monitor screen. A normal heart rhythm looks like spikes and domes at regular intervals.

Automated Blood Pressure Cuff: Squeeze and Release

Your blood pressure is measured with a plastic cuff, which usually is wrapped around your upper arm. Sometimes the cuff is wrapped elsewhere—for example, around your calf if one arm is being operated on and the other arm is not available (broken or burned). The automated blood pressure cuff inflates and deflates at regular intervals set by the anesthesiologist. The first inflation feels the tightest and might be uncomfortable.

A TYPICAL
ELECTROCARDIOGRAM

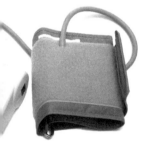

A BLOOD PRESSURE
CUFF

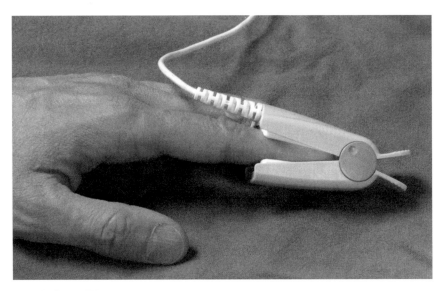

A PULSE OXIMETER

100

A PULSE OXIMETER
TRACING

Automation helps doctors focus on other matters, because a current blood pressure reading will always be on the display monitor. The top number is called the systolic pressure, and the bottom number is the diastolic pressure. The number in parentheses is the mean (average) blood pressure.

Pulse Oximeter: Fingertip Light

The oxygen level in your blood is measured with a pulse oximeter. It is a clip-on or adhesive device, usually attached to your fingertip, that transmits a red light. The pulse oximeter can also be attached to your toe, earlobe, or even your forehead if the signal from your finger is weak.

It's best not to wear nail polish on the day of surgery, because the red light needs to penetrate through layers of your nail and be absorbed in the blood. The pulse oximeter reading appears as a waveform as well as a number. The regularity of the waveform and the number level also correlate with a beeping sound. The higher the oxygen level in your blood, the higher the tone of the beep. The faster your heart rate, the more rapidly the beeping occurs.

Malignant Hyperthermia: An Anesthesia Emergency!

An uncommon genetic defect can make some patients prone to **malignant hyperthermia** (MH). This is a condition of extremely high body temperature that can only be seen when a predisposed person is exposed to anesthetic gases or the muscle relaxant succinylcholine, which are the triggering agents.

A rapid rise in body temperature, muscle rigidity (tightness), dark-colored urine, and abnormal blood chemistry are some of the telltale signs of MH. This is an anesthetic emergency, because the body is essentially boiling up from the inside. Fortunately, there is a standardized treatment for the MH crisis that can save the patient. A medication called dantrolene must be given immediately if an MH crisis is suspected. But dantrolene is only part of the treatment. In addition, introducing cooled fluids, applying ice on the body, supplying 100 percent oxygen, and protecting the heart, brain, and kidneys are essential in

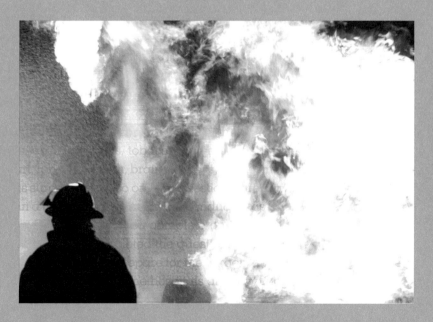

crisis management. Most episodes of MH occur in the operating room, but symptoms can appear in the first few hours after recovery from general anesthesia.

Conservatively, the incidence of malignant hyperthermia is about 1 in 20,000 to 50,000 adults undergoing general anesthesia. The mortality rate from a full-blown attack can be as high as 10 percent. Remember, the chance of occurrence depends on having a genetic defect (1 in 3,000) *and* being exposed to the triggering anesthetics (inhaled gases and succinylcholine). It is not possible to predict if you will have such a crisis unless you know of a close relative with a definite episode of MH or one who has been diagnosed to carry the gene. Furthermore, some medical conditions such as muscular dystrophy (or a history of it in the family) can predispose to MH with triggering drugs. To make things even more challenging, it is possible to have a previous uneventful surgery with general anesthesia and still be at risk for MH. Many people find out about their MH risk after it occurs. There are about a thousand cases reported each year.

Diagnostic tests are available in specialized centers. Muscle biopsy testing is the most sensitive and specific way to determine if you are prone to MH. Genetic testing has also been developed. It is not practical to test every patient before surgery. Anesthesiologists are working on developing rapid DNA analysis tests. *If any family member has had an episode of MH, all other family members, including cousins, should be alerted to their potential risk.* Any person with such complications should register their MH susceptibility with the North American MH Registry of the Malignant Hyperthermia Association of the United States (MHAUS), based in Pennsylvania, by calling toll-free (888) 274-7899. The MHAUS also has an informative Web site: www.mhaus.org.

If you know of any family members with a history of anesthetic deaths or complications, inform your anesthesia provider before undergoing surgery. The anesthesia provider will take special precautions and avoid drugs that can trigger MH. If you are planning to have surgery under general anesthesia (inhaled gas or succinylcholine), these are the questions you can ask:

- Does the facility have dantrolene?
- Does the facility have the capacity to treat an MH crisis?
- Is there an MH kit or cart readily available?

Survival from an MH crisis in a non-hospital location is ensured by rapid transfer to a major medical center.

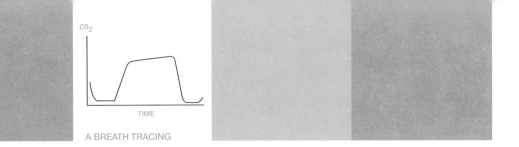

CO₂

TIME

A BREATH TRACING

Capnograph: Every Breath You Take

A **capnograph** measures the amount of carbon dioxide exhaled in every breath. Carbon dioxide is a naturally exhaled gas eliminated from your body. The presence of exhaled carbon dioxide lets the anesthesiologist know that adequate ventilation is taking place. In other words, oxygen is moving *in* and carbon dioxide is moving *out* of your lungs in a regular manner.

The exhaled carbon dioxide (CO_2) is sampled close to the mouth or nose. A breath tracing is a curved or boxed waveform along with a number. It is the best indicator that your air passages are open.

Temperature Sensors: Warm and Toasty

It's important to maintain your normal body temperature during surgery. Normal human body temperature is 37.5 degrees Celsius (98.6 degrees Fahrenheit). During surgery the temperature of the body tends to drop, due to the effects of anesthesia and from exposure to a cold operating room. Keeping your temperature as close to normal is the goal in most surgical procedures.

 *Devices such as **warming blankets** (also called forced-air blankets) and fluid warmers help maintain your temperature near normal. In some types of heart and brain surgery, however, **deliberate hypothermia**, or lowering the body temperature on purpose, is required for a short time to protect the brain.*

To monitor your body temperature when you're under general anesthesia, the anesthesiologist will often insert a soft plastic sensor into your esophagus. In sedated patients, a sensor may be placed in the underarm. The sensor transmits signals to a monitor that displays the temperature reading.

Special Monitors

Some patients require additional monitoring due to the type of surgery they're having. For example, continuous measurement of blood pressure is needed if a large amount of blood loss is anticipated or blood pressure is not stable. Specialized monitors may also be used because of certain underlying health conditions (heart disease, lung disease, kidney disease, obesity, or trauma, for example).

 Keep in mind that the placement of all invasive devices has potential risks as well as benefits. The anesthesiologist uses these monitors when the benefits outweigh the risks. For example, one of the risks of a central line placement in the neck area is a punctured lung—but the central line may be essential in circumstances when direct measurement of the amount of blood filling the heart is needed.

Arterial Line: Measure Blood Pressure Right inside the Body

An **arterial line** is a catheter that allows measurement of your blood pressure on a continuous basis directly from an artery. It is placed under sterile conditions.

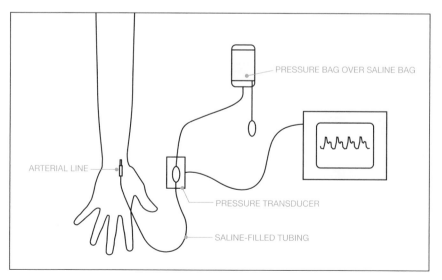

ARTERIAL LINE

PRESSURE BAG OVER SALINE BAG

PRESSURE TRANSDUCER

SALINE-FILLED TUBING

AN ARTERIAL LINE SETUP

The arterial line catheter looks very much like an intravenous (IV) line. It's usually placed on the wrist on the thumb side (radial artery). It could also be placed on the groin (femoral artery), foot (dorsalis pedis artery), or upper arm (axillary artery). If it's placed while you're awake, the area is numbed with local anesthetic to prevent discomfort.

The measurement technique is based on the principle that each heartbeat generates a pulsatile (rhythmic) blood flow in the arteries throughout your body.

Blood samples can be drawn from an arterial line to measure blood gas levels (oxygen, carbon dioxide), acid/base status, blood chemistry (sodium, potassium, and calcium), red blood cell level (hematocrit), and blood sugar (glucose).

Central Line: A Big IV in the Heart

A **central line** is a long catheter placed in your neck veins (internal jugular or subclavian veins) reaching down to the large vessel entering your heart (superior vena cava).

In essence, it's a larger IV line that is always placed under sterile conditions. A central line may be placed while you're awake (with local

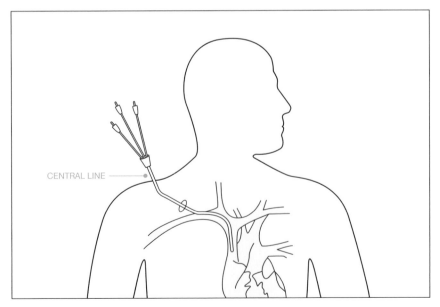

CENTRAL LINE

A CENTRAL LINE IN PLACE

numbing) or after you're under general anesthesia. Once a central line is placed, it can be kept in for several days or replaced if necessary.

A central line can be used to administer medications or large amounts of fluid and to replace blood. Blood samples can also be drawn back from the line. A pressure sensor can be attached to measure the **central venous pressure**. The central venous pressure reflects the amount of blood circulating in the body, and it gives doctors information about how well the heart is working.

Blood Circulation

Blood from throughout the body returns to the heart, entering chambers called the right atrium and then the right ventricle. The right ventricle of the heart pumps blood into the lungs so the blood can be **oxygenated**, or combined with oxygen. The oxygenated blood then enters the left-sided chambers of the heart called the left atrium and left ventricle. The left ventricle pumps blood from the heart throughout the body.

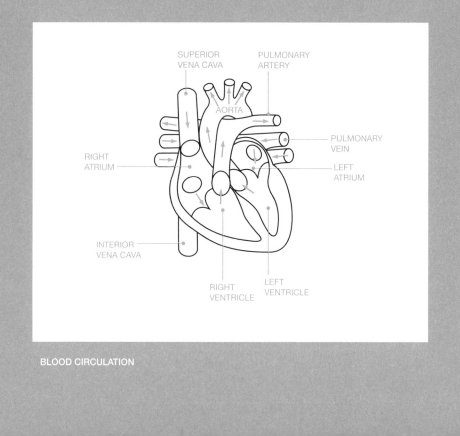

SUPERIOR VENA CAVA

PULMONARY ARTERY

AORTA

PULMONARY VEIN

RIGHT ATRIUM

LEFT ATRIUM

INTERIOR VENA CAVA

RIGHT VENTRICLE

LEFT VENTRICLE

BLOOD CIRCULATION

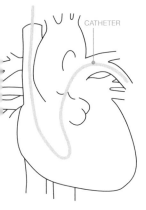

CATHETER

A PULMONARY
ARTERY CATHETER
IN PLACE

Pulmonary Artery Catheter: More about the Heart and Blood Circulation

A **pulmonary artery catheter** (PAC) is a long, thin plastic catheter floated into your heart and up the great blood vessels entering the lungs (through the pulmonary artery). Sometimes it's called a Swan-Ganz catheter in honor of its inventors, Jeremy Swan and William Ganz.

The anesthesiologist introduces the PAC through a large vein in your neck, similar to a central line. As with any other device that enters your body, it is always placed under sterile conditions, either awake with numbing medications or while under general anesthesia.

A PAC is primarily a diagnostic device. It allows doctors to measure the pressure inside the heart chambers and the lung vessels, as well as the amount of blood pumped out of the heart. It also helps to monitor the effects of potent heart and blood pressure medications. A temperature sensor at the tip of the catheter measures blood temperature.

Imaging Monitors

See the Heart in Real Time

The **transesophageal echocardiograph** (TEE) is an imaging device that allows the heart chambers and valves to be pictured on a monitor screen. It is used during heart surgery, for evaluation of heart disease, or during complex surgeries.

While the patient is under general anesthesia, a large probe is placed through the mouth into the esophagus, which lies behind the heart. The TEE uses ultrasound waves, which are transmitted from the tip of the probe. The traveling sound waves bounce off the heart, generating a picture of the pumping heart. The tip of the probe can be moved to show all four chambers of the heart, the heart valves, and the large arteries leaving the heart. The TEE probe provides information about the pumping action of the heart and the amount of blood flowing through the heart.

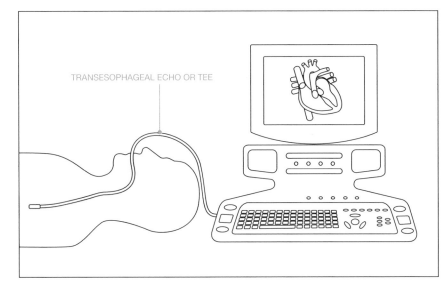

TRANSESOPHAGEAL ECHO OR TEE

A TRANSESOPHAGEAL ECHOCARDIOGRAM (TEE) TAKING PLACE

Brain and Nerve Monitors

Electroencephalograph: Brain Wave Detector

The **electroencephalograph** (EEG) measures the electrical activity of the brain. Although an EEG can be used for many purposes (to identify brain disease or predict the outcome of a brain injury, for example), its main use in anesthesia is during carotid endarterectomy or brain surgery.

The information is obtained by gluing a series of electrodes (sensors) to specific locations on the scalp. The brain signals are picked up by the electrodes and processed by a computer. The information is displayed as a series of irregular waves. The height of the waves, number of waves, and symmetry from both sides of the brain all convey information about brain function.

A person dedicated to interpreting the EEG is in the operating room conveying the information to the anesthesiologist and the surgeon. Actions are taken by the surgeon and anesthesiologist to address any changes in the EEG pattern.

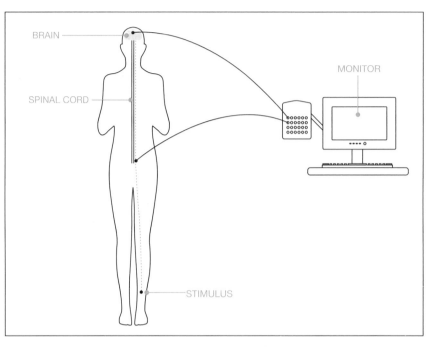

AN EVOKED POTENTIAL SETUP

Evoked Potentials: Keep Nerve Pathways Intact

Evoked potentials are a type of monitoring used in patients having surgery that may place nerve pathways at risk, such as spine surgery. The integrity of these pathways—sensation, movement, hearing, and sight—can be monitored.

Somatosensory evoked potential (SSEP) and motor evoked potential (MEP) are examples of monitoring that may be used during spine surgery. The monitoring helps safeguard the integrity of nerve pathways that control your sensations and movements. A person dedicated to interpreting evoked potentials is in the operating room conveying the information to the anesthesiologist and the surgeon.

As an example for sensory evoked potentials, recording electrodes are placed on the skin over large nerves in the hands and foot, on the back over the spine, and on specific areas of the scalp. A nerve is gently stimulated with an electric current that travels up to the brain. When the brain signal is picked up, it means the pathway from the nerve to the spinal cord and up to the brain is intact and undamaged.

The Sixth Sense: The Best Monitor

You can now appreciate all the equipment that anesthesiologists work with to extend their eyes and ears. Monitors are an extension of a "sixth sense," which is the true skill of anesthesia. The best monitors, though, can't replace an anesthesiologist's ability to anticipate what will happen, plan for it, react appropriately to the unexpected, and learn from the experience.

 Prescriptives: Be a Better Consumer

☐ Notify your anesthesia provider of any problems or complications you have had during previous surgeries. _____

_____

☐ Let the anesthesia provider know if you or any close relative has a history of malignant hyperthermia. _____

_____

☐ Will any special monitors, heart imaging monitors, brain/nerve monitors be used during your surgery?_____

_____

☐ If you are going to have a special monitor placed, how long will it stay in after your surgery? _____

_____

☐ Notify the anesthesia provider if you have experienced any complications with a special monitor in the past. _____

_____

CHAPTERSIX

the recovery room:
wake up and
feel better

Time to wake up from anesthesia! What concerns
you most? Pain? Coming out of surgery in one piece?
How will you feel when you wake up? How long will it
take to feel better?

On the Road Back: Recovery

The recovery room—known to medical people as the
post-anesthesia care unit (PACU)—is a critical-care
area. The word "critical" is emphasized because surgery
changes the body's functions, and anesthesia can have
lingering effects on blood pressure, heart rate, and
breathing.

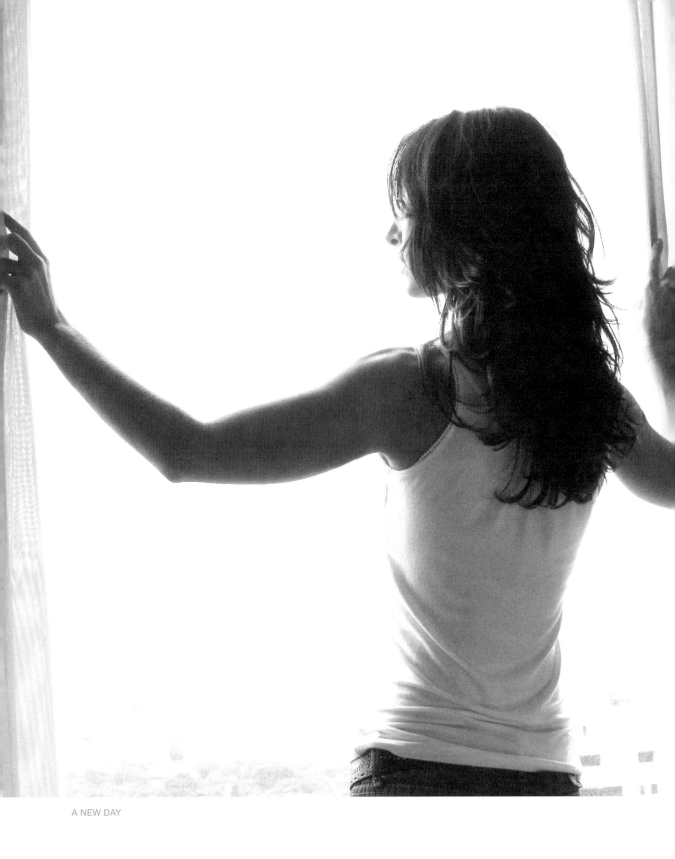

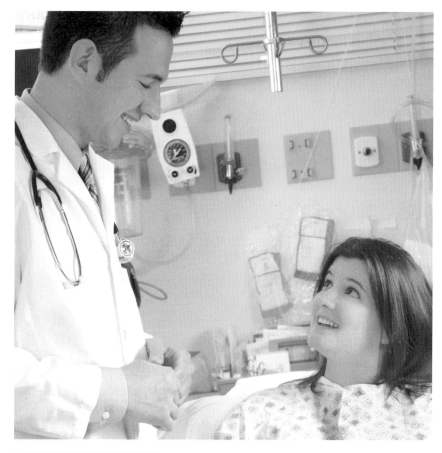

A SMILE MEANS A HAPPY ENDING.

The recovery "room" is actually an open unit with multiple beds. It may have an isolation room. Patients in recovery are under constant vigilance by medical personnel. Usually the ratio is one nurse to two patients. A single nurse is dedicated to a critically ill patient.

Nurses who work in a PACU have a great deal of experience and training in the management of patients after anesthesia. Recovery room nurses have been trained to handle every case—from minor, routine surgical procedures to badly injured trauma victims.

Post-anesthesia care nurses must learn everything they can about each patient. The moment a patient arrives, monitors for heart

rate/rhythm, oxygen level, and blood pressure are attached. (See the description of monitors in chapter 5.) Monitoring with an arterial line or pulmonary artery catheters may be continued or started in the PACU, depending on the needs of the particular patient. The anesthesiologist tells the nurses about the patient's medical history, the type of surgery performed, the type of anesthetic given, any special medications added, and the amount of intravenous (IV) fluid or blood received in the procedure.

Your surgeon and anesthesiologist will work together with your nurse to decide what type of continued care you require. Continued care can mean anything from keeping you on a ventilator, preparing you for extubation (removal of the breathing tube), deciding blood transfusion requirements, controlling blood pressure, minimizing nausea and vomiting, and treating pain, to deciding when you are ready to be discharged.

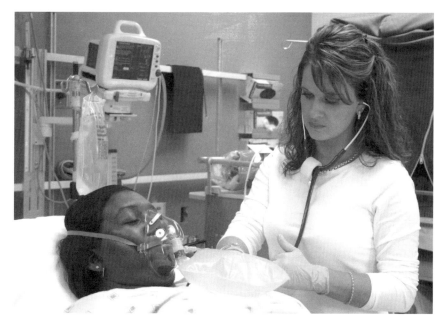

NURSES TAKE CARE OF YOU IN THE RECOVERY ROOM.

Recovery Room Monitoring

In the recovery room, the following are monitored carefully:

- Respiratory system
  - √ Breathing rate
  - √ Airway patency (Is your breathing comfortable?)
  - √ Oxygen level
- Circulatory system
  - √ Pulse rate (Is it too fast or too slow?)
  - √ Heart rhythm (Is it steady and even?)
  - √ Blood pressure (Is it high or low?)
- Muscle strength (Can you move your arms and legs?)
- Consciousness (Are you awake, alert, and oriented to your surroundings?)
- Temperature (Are you hot or cold?)
- Pain level
- Nausea and vomiting control
- Hydration (Is more fluid, less fluid, or blood needed?)
- Color (Is your skin color pink, pale, dusky, or blotchy?)

The purpose of continued monitoring is to make sure that big as well as subtle problems after surgery are detected and acted upon immediately. Problems such as difficulty breathing, decreased oxygen levels, high or low blood pressure, inappropriate heart rate, and an abnormal heart rhythm have to be treated quickly. The PACU nurse will also check your bandages and look for wound drainage or bleeding.

As the anesthesia wears off, you may experience some pain. If this occurs, your nurse will provide additional doses of medication or start a **patient-controlled analgesia** (PCA) device. (This is described in detail in chapter 7.)

Some patients feel cold and shiver uncontrollably when they first wake up after surgery. A mild drop in body temperature is common during general and regional anesthesia, because these drugs alter the body's temperature-regulating abilities. Warm blankets and anti-shivering medications like meperidine (Demerol) are useful at this time.

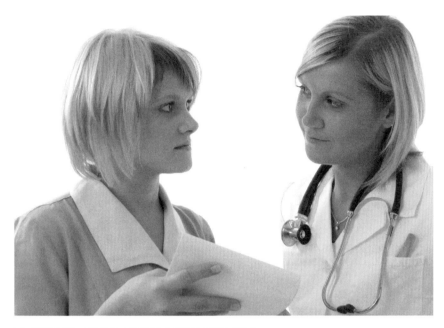

DOCTORS AND NURSES ALWAYS DISCUSS YOUR CARE.

How quickly you recover from anesthesia depends on the type of anesthetic you received (see chapter 2), your individual response to anesthesia, and how fast the medications are cleared from your body. For some people, emerging from general anesthesia causes some confusion and disorientation. A person's age and general health also affect how quickly he recovers. It may take some time before the effects of general anesthesia or sedative medications wear off.

Some effects of anesthesia may last for many hours after a procedure. For example, a general anesthetic may leave you tired and drowsy for the remainder of the day and even into the next day. After a regional anesthetic, there may be continued numbness or weakness for a few hours in the part of the body that was operated on. Patients are monitored for the wearing off of regional anesthesia. Signs that a regional anesthetic is wearing off are a return of sensation and movement in the part of the body that was blocked for surgery. Having difficulty urinating is a common side effect of epidural or spinal anesthesia. As the epidural and spinal medications wear off, the ability to urinate returns.

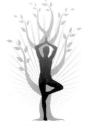

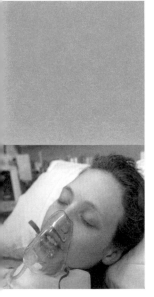

Recovery Room Setups

Recovery rooms are divided into level I and level II areas. The level I area requires patients to remain in bed and be monitored as described above. The level II recovery area allows patients to sit in recliners, walk with assistance, drink fluids, and eat a light snack. The monitoring standards are less rigid in the level II area.

Those patients who need more time in the hospital to recuperate are transferred to floor beds or **intensive care** units (ICUs) directly from the recovery room level I. In a hospital setting, a patient may go directly from the operating room to the level II area, with the anesthesiologist's permission.

Same-day (or ambulatory) surgery procedures have led to changes in anesthetic techniques and the development of short-acting medications that allow for rapid recovery—meaning, as the name of the surgery says, that patients can go home the same day. Today, short-acting anesthetics permit the anesthesiologist to easily have patients up and about and ready for discharge. An office-based surgery practice or independent surgery center has only a level II–type area, so recovery from anesthesia must be quick.

When Can I Get Out of Here?

Unless the surgical team determines that you should be admitted to the hospital overnight, a number of guidelines must be followed before you are considered ready to go home. Recovery and discharge guidelines after a regional anesthetic are the same as for general anesthesia, but they also require a progressive return of sensation and control of movement in the area of the body that was blocked for surgery.

There is no minimal mandatory stay in the recovery room, because each person recovers differently. Patients are watched until they are no longer at risk of side effects from anesthesia and there is no apparent complication. Before leaving the hospital, you will be given instructions about your diet, medications, and activities—and a phone number to call in case of emergency.

Discharge Guidelines

Here are some broad discharge guidelines followed by many surgical facilities:

- Your vital signs (heart rate, oxygen level, and blood pressure) have stabilized to the range they were in before your procedure.
- Your consciousness and mental status have returned to their pre-surgical levels.
- You appear to be calm and comfortable.
- Any nausea and vomiting is under control.
- Your pain control is considered at a "tolerable level."
- Your ability to move about is consistent with your age and general health status.
- You have progressively returning sensory and motor control of your arms and legs (after regional anesthesia).
- Your ability to urinate is documented (some centers require this).
- You have an escort who will take you directly home and stay with you in case you need to return to the hospital.

What can be expected after you get home? For most patients, tiredness is common. In adults, general anesthesia can cause **post-operative nausea and vomiting**. Pain is also common. It is usually the main reason for contacting the surgeon before the next planned follow-up office visit.

Recovery depends on being well informed, planning ahead, and getting lots of rest before and after a procedure. Make sure that the person looking after you has the address and the phone number of your pharmacy so you can have your prescriptions filled. That person should also be informed of the proper dosing of your medications.

Recovery begins in the hospital or other surgical center, but it continues at home. Positive thoughts are an important part of a speedy recovery. The support of friends and family during this time is always a plus. Focus on making small improvements each day, with an eye toward

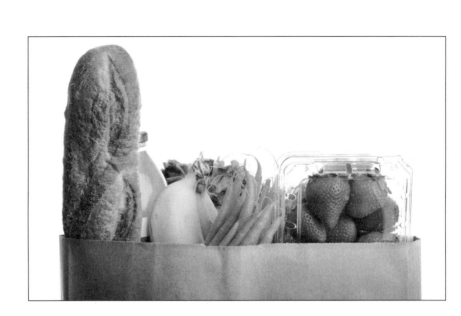

EAT HEALTHY.

continued progress. Your body needs time to heal. Some unexpected setbacks may happen, but a positive attitude will help rebuild your strength.

Don't push yourself or have unrealistic goals. Recovery from surgery has a lot to do with your underlying physical condition before surgery. A young and physically active person is likely to recover faster than an older, frail, inactive person or someone with multiple health problems.

Besides keeping a positive attitude, eat a well-balanced diet, get plenty of rest, and gradually increase physical activity. This will be your path to a new beginning. Congratulate yourself for a job well done!

Now that you are familiar with the setting and routine of the recovery room, you can be more relaxed about what will happen to you after a procedure or surgery. The recovery room is a place to begin healing. This is where you are pampered and coddled after going through an important life experience. That experience may have been a routine procedure (colonoscopy), a required surgery (heart bypass), or something you decided you want (facelift). Whatever the reason you end up in the recovery room, rest assured that it is governed by structure and protocol to ensure your safety.

Dr. Dhar Advises: Take It Easy

Don't plan to drive home from the hospital or off-site surgery center by yourself! A controlled study looked at whether driving alertness had been restored to normal by two and then twenty-four hours after general anesthesia in patients who had same-day surgery. Patients showed impaired driving skills (attention lapses and lower alertness level) two hours after the surgery but were safe to drive twenty-four hours after general anesthesia.

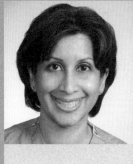

Rx Prescriptives: Be a Better Consumer

☐ Where will you be recovering after surgery—in the recovery room? In the intensive care unit? At home? Ask your doctor. _____

_____

☐ Will you need special monitors (arterial line, central line, pulmonary artery catheter) in the recovery room? _____

_____

☐ Will you be on a ventilator in the recovery room? _____

_____

☐ Once in the recovery room, when will you get to see your loved ones? _____

_____

☐ Is there someone to accompany you home after surgery? Who? _____

_____

☐ Is there someone to take care of you when you get home? Who? _____

_____

CHAPTERSEVEN

the "ouch" factor: controlling pain

Ouch! Scraping your knee is painful. Bumping your funny bone on the edge of the table hurts. Even touching a hot cup of coffee can be painful. Pain can be caused by anything that invades the integrity of your skin, internal organs, and bones. After a surgical or diagnostic procedure, pain is defined as an unpleasant sensation of varying degree and character resulting from changes in the integrity of the body.

IMAGINE A SOFT LANDING.

People instinctively shy away from pain whenever possible, but pain is a complex protective mechanism. Everything from a little paper cut to a broken arm reminds us of our fragility.

After an injury, we take steps to protect ourselves, learn from the experience, and avoid repeating the situation. Pain, then, helps us learn what to avoid.

Pain Protects You—Really!

A complex network of nerve endings, chemical transmitters, the spinal cord, and the brain is responsible for how you perceive your surroundings. Specialized sensory nerve endings called **nociceptors** can be

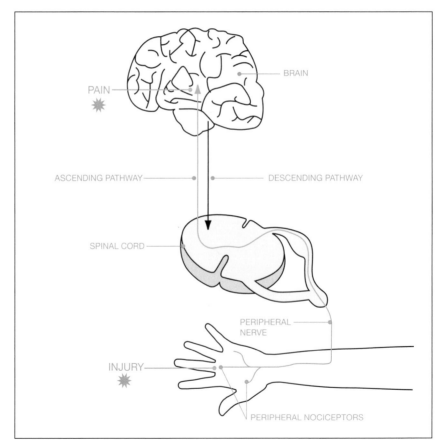

A PAIN PATHWAY

found throughout the body. Nociceptors detect sensations such as hot, cold, sharpness, and pressure. The information from these nerve endings travels to your spinal cord and then to your brain. In the brain, the information is perceived, processed, and reacted upon.

Say you accidentally touch a hot iron with your hand. The nerve signal travels from the nociceptors in your hand to the spine and then to your brain, where the information is quickly analyzed. The brain then sends back the message to take your hand away from the heat—now! This whole process takes only a second or so.

The protective value of pain can be seen in a rare genetic disorder known as congenital insensitivity to pain. Patients with this disorder have abnormal responses to pain. These may range from an inability to describe the intensity or type of pain, to not flinching and withdrawing from something painful. You might think that life without pain would be wonderful. But without experiencing pain, consider all the major injuries you could have that would threaten your very being!

Who's Complaining, Anyway?

Pain often causes emotional reactions, ranging from mild annoyance to sadness, anger, depression, or even fear. How people react emotionally to pain is very personal and individual.

Our physical reactions to pain can be either involuntary or voluntary. Most people will automatically jerk their hand away from a hot object. That's an example of an involuntary reaction. But there's another type of reaction to pain, known as voluntary reaction. Examples are putting a bandage on a cut and asking someone for help in relieving the sting of a burn from touching a hot frying pan.

Voluntary reactions are influenced by your personality (how you deal with pain), your expectations of how sympathetic others will be, and social, cultural, and environmental factors.

⚠️ *People react differently to pain. Some of us are more sensitive to pain than others. For example, some women find that early labor pain is unbearable, while others can wait longer before requesting an epidural. And, of course, some women choose to "tough it out" without any pain-relief medication at all. Some people have a high tolerance level to pain; others have a low tolerance level.*

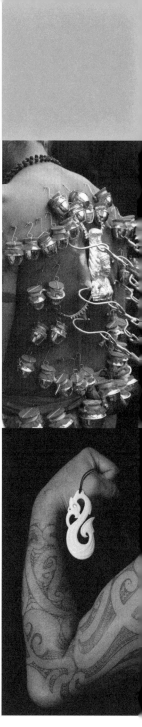

GETTING TATTOOS OR PIERCINGS MAY TEST YOUR PAIN TOLERANCE.

Just the thought of hurting may heighten the sensitivity to pain in someone who is awaiting surgery.

Depending on the situation or the environment you're in, you can expect a different reaction to your display of pain. For example, you can expect more sympathy from a doctor or nurse in the hospital than from a tough army sergeant in basic training. This expected reaction from those around you may influence how you behave and deal with pain.

Different cultures have different attitudes and responses toward pain. People in some cultures are stoic—they outwardly show little or no reaction to pain—while people in other cultures are thought to be quite dramatic in how they express pain. Even different religions have different expectations and beliefs about pain. All of these influences play a part in how you perceive and react to pain.

Put on a Happy Face

In our society, the modern approach toward pain is to control it aggressively in all age groups. Heightened pain delays the healing process and clouds a sense of control over the body. Other negative effects of pain include increased blood pressure and heart rate, which are especially bad for people with heart disease. Pain-control medications and the devices that deliver them are widely available for all age groups, including newborns. The importance of pain control has made pain management a part of anesthesiology.

WONG-BAKER FACES PAIN RATING SCALE

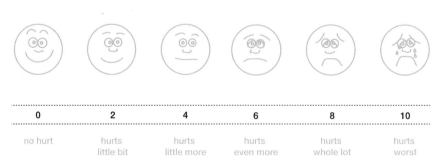

0	2	4	6	8	10
no hurt	hurts little bit	hurts little more	hurts even more	hurts whole lot	hurts worst

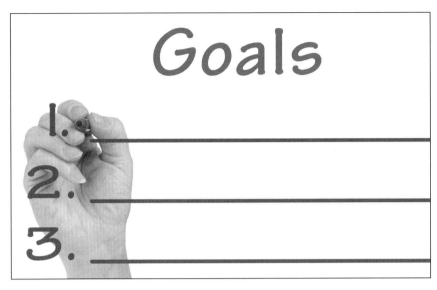

THINK OF YOUR GOALS AFTER SURGERY.

Before a procedure, be sure to discuss the plan for pain control with your surgeon and your anesthesiologist. Tell them about your experiences with pain so that they have a better understanding of the level of your sensitivity and tolerance.

Your anesthesia provider may assess your pain by asking you to indicate a level on the visual rating scale (VRS) or visual analog scale (VAS). Ten, or a sad face, is considered the worst imaginable pain; zero, or a happy face, means you feel no pain at all. The obvious goal in pain management is for you to point to zero.

Taking Control: Pain Medication

Pain medications work at the level of the nerves, spinal cord, and brain either by blocking the nerve signal or by distorting the interpretation of these signals by the brain. Sometimes combinations of medications can be more helpful than a single drug. Research on new medications and treatments are changing the way anesthesiologists manage pain. Let's look at some of the common types of pain medication you can expect after a procedure or surgery.

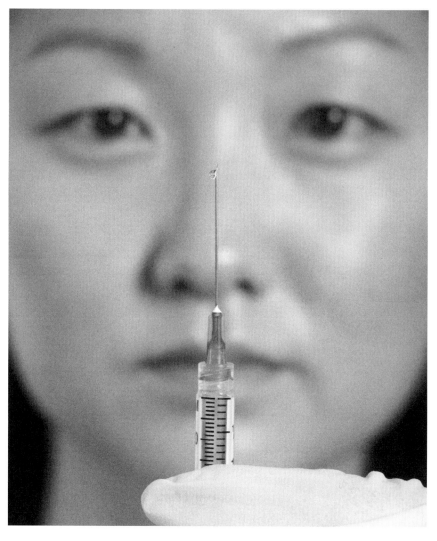

YIKES! THE FEWER OF THESE, THE BETTER.

Non-steroidal Anti-inflammatory Drugs (NSAIDs)

The most popular non-steroidal anti-inflammatory drugs (NSAIDs) are aspirin, ibuprofen (Motrin, Advil), and naproxen (Aleve). NSAIDs reduce pain, inflammation, and fever. Skin and musculoskeletal pain usually respond to these drugs. Ketorolac (Toradol) is a potent NSAID that can be given in the operating room at the end of surgery. A single dose of ketorolac (15 to 30 milligrams) is equivalent to a few milligrams of morphine, a powerful narcotic (**opioid**).

 NSAIDS increase the risk of bleeding because they block the action of platelets (blood cells), which are essential for clotting.

Acetaminophen

Acetaminophen, popularly known as Tylenol, is an excellent pain reliever and fever reducer. It has no anti-inflammatory effect.

Acetaminophen is a component of many over-the-counter drugs and prescription combinations, including propoxyphene-acetaminophen (Darvocet) and oxycodone-acetaminophen (Percocet).

 There is a risk of liver damage if the recommended dose of acetaminophen is exceeded or an acute overdose is taken. (The maximum daily dose is 4 grams in adults and 75 milligrams per kilogram in children.) Certain patients, such as people who abuse alcohol, may be at risk of liver damage at a lower dose.

Opioids (Narcotics)

Opioids are also called **narcotics**. Opioids alter the way in which pain signals are interpreted by the brain and spinal cord.

Morphine is the "gold standard" for this category—that is, the potency (strength) of all the other narcotics is compared to morphine. A few well-known drug names in this category are oxycodone (Oxycontin), hydrocodone (Vicodin), meperidine (Demerol), fentanyl, and tramadol (Ultram). Opioids vary in their potency and duration of action (how long they're effective).

Anesthesiologists use opioids in many ways. For example, a small dose of fentanyl can be injected into the spinal or epidural space (areas surrounding the spinal cord) to provide continued effective pain control after abdominal or lower body surgery.

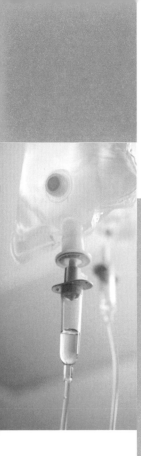

⚠️ *Some possible side effects resulting from the use of opioids are nausea, vomiting, drowsiness, itching, constipation, and euphoria (sense of well-being). Not all patients experience such effects. There is no dosage limit on a particular opioid unless the side effects of excessive sedation or decreased breathing rate occur.*

Risky Pain Killer: Methadone

Methadone has become popular as a medication for hard-to-treat pain conditions: joint pain, back pain, and a variety of other pains not easily relieved by non-narcotic drugs.

But methadone is tricky, and if not used properly it can lead to death. It is the fastest-growing cause of narcotic deaths in the United States. The reason is that every person reacts differently to methadone. That is, the absorption, metabolism, and response are individualized. If methadone is mixed with alcohol or other sedative medications, a person's breathing rate can drop down to zero.

It is important for people to stay under the care of a physician, and perhaps even a pain specialist, when taking methadone. Doctors have to be extra-vigilant during the start of treatment, during conversion from one opioid drug to another, and during dose increases.

Let your anesthesia provider know if you have taken methadone, because it stays in the body for a long time. Certain anesthetic drugs can add to its sedative effect.

Local Anesthetics

Local anesthetics block transmission of pain impulses from the nerves to the spinal cord and brain. These agents can be injected into a body cavity, around nerves, or directly into a surgical incision. What's more, cocaine is occasionally used as a local anesthetic in the nose (for nasal intubation or nasal surgery)!

⚠ *Each local anesthetic has a dosage limit. Doses that are poisonous— toxic—may lead to abnormal heart rhythms, decreased breathing, light-headedness, difficulty focusing, ringing in the ears, changes in oxygen binding to blood cells (methemoglobinemia), and seizures.*

PanchLines

Dr. Dhar Suggests: Think of Alternatives

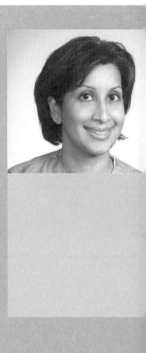

There are natural ways to relieve acute pain that do not involve pre-scribed medications or medical procedures. These methods are not for everyone, but they have gained in popularity as adjuncts for healing. Proper nutrition, rest, and regular exercise allow a broader approach to health and healing. Here are some other approaches you can add to your recovery. Consult your doctor before taking supplements along with your regular medication.

- A homeopathic remedy such as arnica can help with healing of bruises and swelling.
- Vitamins such as A, C, E, thiamine (B1), and pantothenic acid (B5) may reduce wound healing time and enhance tissue strength.
- A cream containing small amounts of capsaicin, the active in-gredient of cayenne pepper, can temporarily relieve pain when rubbed over arthritic joints and areas of muscle pain. It works by depleting sensory nerves of a pain-mediating chemical transmitter known as substance P.
- Bromelain supplements may reduce swelling, bruising, inflam-mation, and pain after surgery and injury. Bromelain is a mix-ture of enzymes found naturally in the juice and stems of pineapples.
- Nutritional supplements containing glucosamine and chondroitin sulfate stimulate production of joint cartilage, leading to improved joint function and reduced pain.

Popular Techniques for Pain Management after a Procedure

The control of pain after surgery or another medical procedure is an important part of recovery and healing. A well-planned approach can make a difference in your overall experience. The anesthesiologist can explain the details of each pain management plan and help you choose what is best for you.

Patient-Controlled Analgesia

Patient-controlled analgesia (PCA) lets you control when you receive pain medication. With PCA, a medication-dispensing pump is attached to an IV line or epidural catheter.

The pump is mounted to a pole near the hospital bed. When the patient pushes a demand button, a fixed amount of medication (called a **bolus**) is delivered on an as-needed basis. A **lockout interval** is a

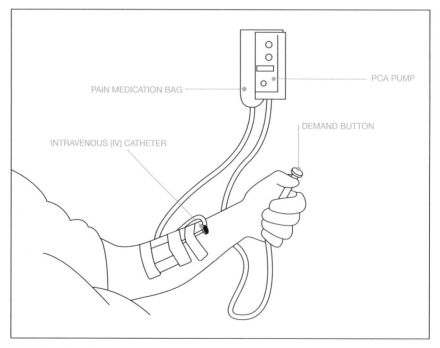

PAIN MEDICATION BAG

PCA PUMP

DEMAND BUTTON

INTRAVENOUS (IV) CATHETER

A PATIENT-CONTROLLED ANALGESIA SETUP

predetermined time that prevents repeated dosing even if you press the demand button. This prevents an overdose of medication. The pump can also be programmed to deliver a low-dose continuous amount of medication in addition to the demand doses. All three settings—continuous dose, demand dose, and lockout interval—can be changed based on your needs. Before being released from the hospital, you will be weaned from the PCA device and given oral medication to control pain.

Intravenous patient-controlled analgesia (IVPCA) allows only an opioid to be delivered. Epidural patient-controlled analgesia (EPCA) permits an opioid and/or a local anesthetic to be delivered.

Here are some of the advantages of PCA:

- You feel less anxious because *you have control* over when you get medication.
- Limited doses prevent an overdose or addiction.
- No need to wait for a nurse to give you pain medication.
- No more repeated shots.
- No need to swallow multiple pills.
- Smaller and more frequent doses mean less sleepiness and weakness.
- Around-the-clock consistent pain control.
- Set dose intervals reduce the overall amount of medication needed.
- You can self-dose to control pain before movement (for example, before physical therapy or getting out of bed).

Continuous Peripheral Nerve Block

A thin plastic catheter can be placed through the skin directly next to a nerve leading to a surgical site, the area that was operated on. The catheter is connected to a pump for supplying local anesthetic, providing site-specific pain control. This technique, known as a **continuous peripheral nerve block**, is popular in orthopedic surgery.

In some medical centers, ambulatory (same-day surgery) patients can go home with the catheter connected to a small, lightweight, disposable pump. This technique is becoming increasingly popular, and ongoing research studies are advancing pump delivery systems.

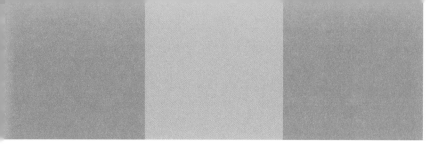

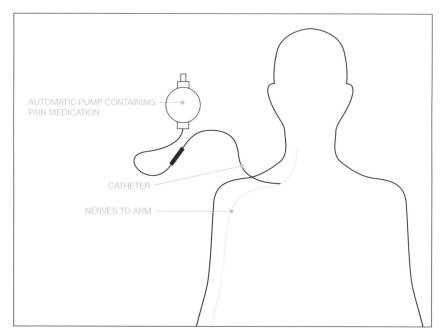

AUTOMATIC PUMP CONTAINING
PAIN MEDICATION

CATHETER

NERVES TO ARM

A CONTINUOUS PERIPHERAL NERVE BLOCK SETUP

Here are some of the advantages of a continuous peripheral nerve block:

- It provides long-lasting pain control with fewer side effects compared to oral or IV medications. This means less nausea, vomiting, itching, sedation, and constipation.
- It significantly lowers pain scores compared to using only oral medication. This means fewer awakenings from sleep because of pain.
- Earlier discharge from the hospital is possible. This means there is less chance of getting an infection in the hospital—which can lead to an overall cost savings for you.

Special Concerns: Addiction Relapse after Anesthesia?

Here's an important question: Do the drugs used during and after anesthesia trigger relapse in former addicts regardless of how long they've been off drugs or alcohol?

Patients recovering from addiction may be extra anxious about anesthesia and concerned about the possibility of relapse. They may also fear that their pain will not be treated completely because of their history of addiction.

Heroin and prescription painkillers such as oxycodone, oxymorphone, hydrocodone, and hydromorphone belong to a category of drugs called opioids, or narcotics. Although opioids are the tried-and-true panacea for pain relief, they are certainly addictive if misused.

It is very important that drug use is mentioned to the anesthesiologist before surgery. Substitute drugs such as methadone and buprenorphine (Suboxone, Subutex) are taken by people recovering from opioid addiction to prevent withdrawal symptoms. The anesthesiologist may instruct the patient to take the daily methadone dose the morning of surgery or decide to give an equivalent intravenous dose during surgery.

⚠️ *Not revealing information about alcohol and illicit drug use does affect anesthetic care. The anesthesiologist may notice the patient requires more than the usual doses of anesthesia. Also, not knowing about opioid use may lead doctors to give lower doses of pain medication during and after surgery. This can lead to inadequate pain control after surgery. Withdrawal can set in if the patient does not have access to alcohol or a drug substitute.*

Thankfully, modern anesthesia is not one size fits all. Nowadays it's tailored to the patient. Here are some things for anyone recovering from opioid (pain reliever) addiction to discuss with the anesthesiologist:

- Can a *lower dose* of opioids be used, or can opioids be completely *avoided* for brief sedation (twilight sleep)?

- Can a lower dose of opioids be used *during* general anesthesia or *held off* until the end of surgery, for post-surgical pain control?
- Can spinal, epidural, peripheral nerve block, or local anesthesia be used *during* surgery?
- Can these regional techniques be used for pain control *after* surgery?
- Can pain medications such as ketorolac (Toradol) that have no abuse potential be used for pain relief?
- Can PCA (patient-controlled analgesia) be used for pain control?

Recovery from drug or alcohol addiction is more than just stopping taking drugs or alcohol. Behavioral changes and social support networks are also essential for staying healthy. Surgery is not the time to undergo detox and rehab.

Rapid Drug Detox under Anesthesia?

Many Web sites advertise an "ultra" rapid drug detox under anesthesia. It sounds like a quick-fix alternative to the traditional detox and rehab programs. The programs using anesthesia essentially let the chemically dependent person sleep through the painful withdrawal symptoms of codeine, heroin, morphine, and other opioid addictions. The idea is to give a person a heavy dose of opioid blockers while they are under general anesthesia. When they awaken, they are already detoxed! Days of painful withdrawal are cut down to hours. The Web sites claim that detoxification is almost 100 percent successful in anesthetized patients.

Sounds like a miracle, but there are dangers involved. This technique does not prevent continued withdrawal symptoms afterwards. Complications such as life-threatening heart rhythm disturbances, fluid in the lungs, stroke, and even death have been reported. Dropout from maintenance treatment can still occur.

What is more, long-term studies have shown that anesthesia-assisted detox is *no more effective* than traditional methods of rehab followed by abstinence.

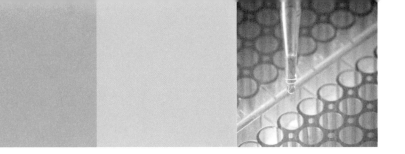

Pain Control in the Future

As in other areas of medicine, pain control is an evolving field. Research on the role of genetics in pain tolerance is being conducted, and scientists have learned that genes can affect an individual's response to certain pain medications. This is why there is a difference between individuals in dosage requirements for pain relief. In the future, pain control may be tailored to a person's genetic profile. So when you sit down with your anesthesia provider to discuss your family background and your medical history, you may find yourself discussing more than the highs and lows of your blood pressure readings.

Pain from any source is something we can all live without. Certainly, pain is a real entity after an operation. But it doesn't have to be inevitable or cripple your quality of life. This chapter has described the standard of care and the new technologies that are helping combat pain after surgery. You can now discuss with your doctor the best pain-treatment approach for you.

Rx **Prescriptives:** Be a Better Consumer

 What is the plan for pain control after your procedure? Be sure to discuss this with your doctor. _____

_____

 Think about your pain tolerance level—is it low, medium, or high? _____

_____

 Have you considered alternative pain relief methods such as relaxation techniques, rest, acupressure, or acupuncture? _____

_____

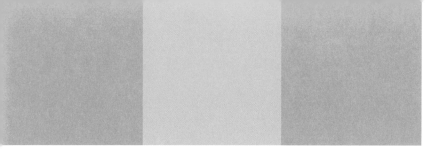

☐ Have you let the anesthesia provider know about all the medications you take regularly? Some medicines interact with pain medicines. _____

_____

☐ Have you told the anesthesia provider about any regular drug use and about how much alcohol you consume? It's especially important to let the anesthesia provider know if you are addicted or think you are addicted to any drugs or alcohol. _____

_____

_____

special topics {

CHAPTEREIGHT {

nips and tucks:
repair, restore, rejuvenate

Are you self-conscious about your sagging jaw-line or stubborn love handles? Does the size of your breasts bother you? Would a nose job help you breathe more easily or correct the disfigurement from a car accident?

If so, maybe you're ready for a nip-and-tuck procedure—and you won't be alone. Every year, millions of people undergo procedures to repair, restore, and rejuvenate their bodies. **Plastic surgery** has come to the forefront in the wonderful world of self-improvement. The aging population and an increasing number of teenagers are

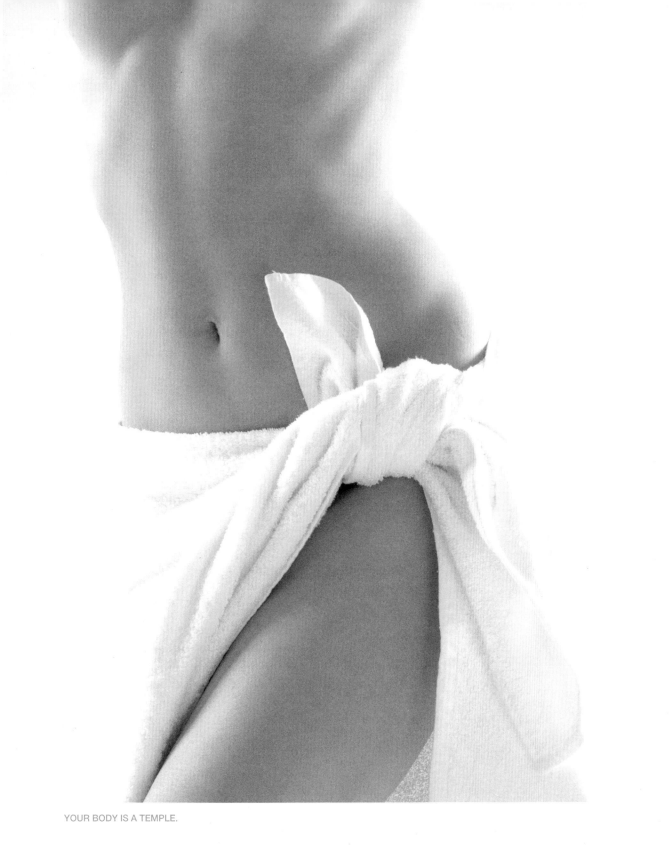

YOUR BODY IS A TEMPLE.

choosing to have aesthetic enhancement. Some 11.8 million cosmetic procedures were performed in the United States in 2007. Of those procedures, 1.1 million were performed on men. The number is expected to increase each year.

Learn the Terms

When we think of plastic surgery, what we usually mean is **cosmetic surgery**—an elective surgery for the sole purpose of improving and modifying one's appearance. Cosmetic surgery is different from **reconstructive plastic surgery**, which is done to improve function and approximate a normal appearance from the effects of trauma (such as a laceration repair after a car accident), acquired defects (burn scars), birth defects (cleft palate), or physical needs (breast reduction). The world of plastic surgery includes both cosmetic and reconstructive surgery.

There is some overlap in the terms, because in most procedures the aesthetic (relating to perceived beauty/appearance) and functional components are not mutually exclusive.

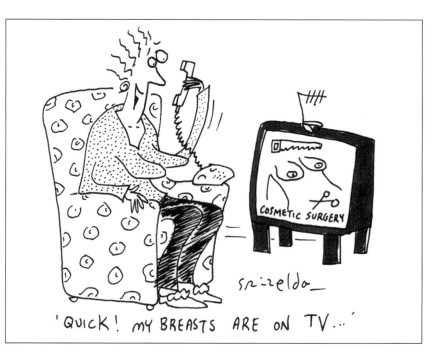

The Standards of "Beauty"

What exactly is "beauty"? The definition and perceptions change with the times. In the 1950s, the actress Marilyn Monroe set the standard for beauty in the United States—curvaceous, soft and rounded, with generous hips and breasts. In the 2000s, big breasts (sometimes eye-poppingly big!) remain popular. But otherwise, a very lean, angular, muscular body type is generally considered to be *the* standard of beauty for women today. Among men, "six-pack abs" are coveted and many have ramped up the wish list. They now want "eight-packs"!

Each person is different, though. Try not to be swayed by the beauty standard *du jour*. Keep in mind what *you* think is beautiful on *you*.

Images in the media have a huge influence on our thinking of what constitutes "beautiful." Television shows such as *Nip/Tuck* and *Dr. 90210* have glamorized the lives of cosmetic surgeons and the results for their patients. Fashion and gossip magazines routinely feature articles on the latest trends and techniques in cosmetic surgery. Many of the celebrities we read about have surgically modified their looks.

New surgical techniques are making cosmetic surgery safer, quicker, cheaper, and more accessible to the average person. This chapter guides you through the process.

What's Hot

Top Cosmetic Procedures for Women
- Breast augmentation
- Liposuction
- Eyelid surgery
- Tummy tuck
- Breast reduction

Top Cosmetic Procedures for Men
- Liposuction
- Eyelid surgery
- Nose reshaping
- Male breast reduction
- Hair transplantation

Source: The American Society for Aesthetic Plastic Surgery, 2007 data

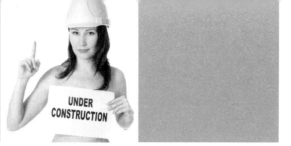

Prepare for Your Transformation

Before you decide to have cosmetic surgery, remember that you must follow the same safeguards you would apply to any surgical procedure. Informed medical consent documents and pre- and post-procedure instructions should be given to you ahead of time.

 As with any surgical procedure, you need to be completely up front with your surgeon and anesthesiologist about any health issues and lifestyle habits that you have.

Not all cosmetic procedures require anesthesia. But the following steps illustrate some things you should consider when planning to have a procedure that will involve anesthesia.

Get to Know Your Surgeon

Qualified plastic surgeons, dermatologic surgeons, otolaryngologists (ear, nose, and throat specialists), maxillofacial (mouth and face) surgeons, and ocular (eye) plastic surgeons are the doctors who perform cosmetic procedures.

Before choosing a surgeon, do your research. Here are some facts to investigate:

- Is the doctor a board-certified physician?
- Is the doctor a member of a leading professional organization (for example, the American Society for Aesthetic Plastic Surgery)?
- Where did the surgeon train in *cosmetic* surgery (not just general surgery)?
- How many procedures of the same type has the doctor performed?
- Will this surgeon you initially consulted with do the procedure personally? If not, what are the qualifications of the other medical professionals?

Ask about Your Anesthesia Provider

It's important to find out about your anesthesia plan, the possible alternatives, and the risks and benefits of each plan. Even cosmetic surgery, which is elective, is still *surgery*. So you must make sure that the people who will be part of the surgery are well qualified for the specific procedure.

Here are some questions that you must answer before undergoing any procedure:

- Is the anesthesia provider a board-certified physician (anesthesiologist)? Or will your anesthesia be delivered by a certified registered nurse anesthetist (CRNA)?
- Is a pre-anesthesia evaluation performed before the procedure?
- Will you meet the anesthesia provider on the day of surgery, or beforehand?

Be Realistic

A health evaluation is required before cosmetic surgery, because not everyone is a good candidate. A person may have a very strong desire to get liposuction, but if he is in poor physical condition—for example, a heavy smoker with poorly controlled heart disease and diabetes—he may be at increased risk of complications from surgery and anesthesia.

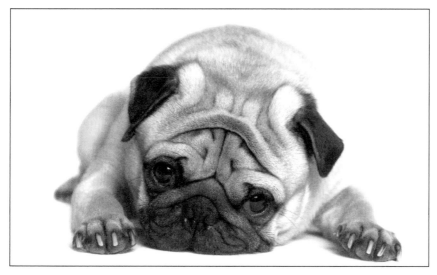

WRINKLES ARE WAITING FOR ALL OF US.

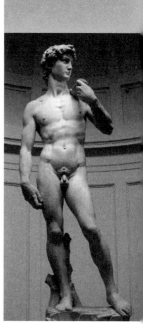

MICHELANGELO'S *DAVID*—AN ENDURING SYMBOL OF MALE BEAUTY

Anesthetic drugs affect all the organ systems of the body. The bodily changes rendered by the anesthetic can place an additional stress on an already weakened heart, lungs, and kidneys. This is especially true for procedures requiring general anesthesia or a prolonged "multiple procedures at one time" situation. The bottom line is . . . persons who are of ASA status 3 should strongly consider not having extensive cosmetic surgery in a non-hospital setting (see chapter 2 for ASA status explanation).

Remember, optimizing your health condition before the scalpel is part of improving your life, too.

⚠️ *Cosmetic surgery is a procedure that you choose to have, not one that is medically necessary. It's important to have realistic expectations about what any cosmetic surgery can do for you.*

Research studies have noted that most people are satisfied with the body part they had surgery on because of improved body image. But there is also data in the other direction—when cosmetic surgery does *not* boost a person's self-esteem, quality of life, self-confidence, and interpersonal relationships in the long term. Basically, don't expect the surgery to change your life!

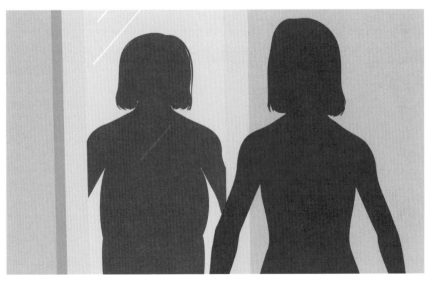

WHAT WE SEE IN THE MIRROR MAY NOT MATCH REALITY.

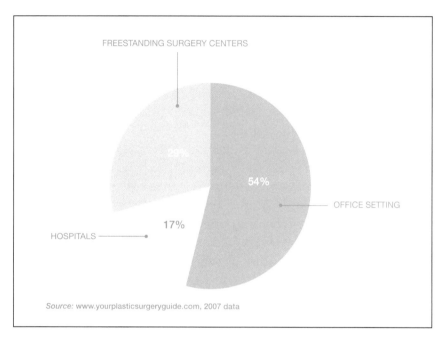

FREESTANDING SURGERY CENTERS

29%

54%

OFFICE SETTING

17%

HOSPITALS

Source: www.yourplasticsurgeryguide.com, 2007 data

WHERE ARE PEOPLE HAVING COSMETIC SURGERY?

Consider the Setting before Signing Up

Cosmetic surgery is done in hospitals, surgery centers, and office-based facilities. About 54 percent of cosmetic procedures are performed in office-based facilities, 29 percent in surgical centers, and 17 percent in hospitals.

Hospital operating rooms have standardized guidelines for equipment and personnel. A non-hospital setting should also have guidelines and be prepared to manage all emergencies, both surgical and anesthetic. The American Society of Anesthesiology has issued standards for office-based anesthesia to ensure your safety during surgery. Research studies have found non-hospital sites to be just as safe as surgery in hospitals. In addition, non-hospital ambulatory (same-day surgery) sites are less expensive, giving more people access to cosmetic procedures. These settings also provide a more private and less stressful environment.

Whatever setting you prefer, make sure that the facility has an *active* **accreditation** by one of the following associations to ensure proper standards of care:

- American Association for Accreditation of Ambulatory Surgery Facilities (AAAASF): (888) 545-5222; www.aaaasf.org
- Accreditation Association for Ambulatory Healthcare (AAAHC): (847) 853-6060; www.aaahc.org
- Joint Commission: (630) 792-5000; www.jointcommission.org
- American Osteopathic Association (AOA): (800) 621-1773; www.osteopathic.org
- Canadian Association for Accreditation of Ambulatory Surgery Facilities (CAAASF): (905) 831-5804; www.caaasf.org
- State department of health (for your state)

Accreditation means that an ambulatory surgery facility meets national standards for equipment, operating safety, personnel, and surgeon credentials. Patients can have confidence that a third party has evaluated the facility and that it has met nationally recognized standards for quality. Accreditation by the AAAASF is recognized as the gold standard. In fact, it is accepted by state departments of health in lieu of state licensing.

Since 2005, the American Board of Facial Plastic and Reconstructive Surgeons (ABFPRS) requires its new members to perform surgery in accredited facilities only.

The following points can help ensure quality and safety in the actual location where a procedure is planned:

- The facility should comply with local, state, and federal regulations. These include laws that protect your health and privacy as a patient. Examples of protective laws are the Occupational Safety and Health Administration (OSHA) blood-borne pathogens (bacteria and viruses) standards and hazardous waste standards, the Americans with Disabilities Act (ADA), and the Health Insurance Portability and Accountability Act (HIPAA).
- Surgeons must be certified (or eligible for certification) by their respective board organizations such as surgery, dermatology,

ophthalmology, otolaryngology (ENT), or oral/maxillofacial surgery. These certificates are usually on display in the doctor's office. The surgeons should have privileges to perform the same surgical procedures in an accredited hospital that is located within thirty minutes of a facility.

- The other personnel assisting in surgery or providing care in the recovery room can't just be anybody. They should be specially trained and certified surgical technicians, registered nurses, and licensed nurse practitioners.
- The equipment must include up-to-date vital sign monitors for procedures requiring more than a topical or strictly local anesthesia. Old or defective devices can mean problems for you.
- Anesthetics such as general anesthesia, spinal anesthesia, epidural anesthesia, or propofol sedation should only be provided by a board-certified or board-eligible anesthesiologist or a CRNA.
- If major surgery is done in a facility, the operating area should be equipped with anesthetic delivery systems, oxygen tanks, vital sign monitors, airway management tools (masks, laryngoscope, endotracheal tube, and so on), and a crash cart.

To learn more, go to www.aaaasf.org.

Crash Cart

A *crash cart* is a portable cart containing emergency resuscitation equipment for patients who are "coding" (when heart rate, heart rhythm, oxygen levels, and blood pressure are in a dangerous range). The emergency equipment includes a **defibrillator** (shock paddles), airway intubation devices, resuscitation bag/mask, and life-saving medication.

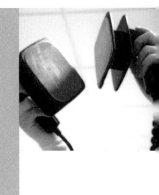

Decide on the Anesthesia

In any cosmetic surgery, the choice of anesthesia is as important as the choice of surgeon, the cost, and the expected result.

⚠️ *Remember, every time an invasive procedure is done, some form of anesthesia is given. An invasive procedure is one in which part of the body is entered by a skin incision or puncture. Breast implants, a facelift, nose reshaping, and liposuction are examples of invasive procedures.*

You may have done hours of research on the type of procedure you're going to have, and you may have decided upon a particular cosmetic surgeon. Now you're excited about becoming the new you. But do you know what type of anesthesia is planned? And who is the anesthesia provider responsible for your comfort and safety?

Cosmetic surgery can be done under local anesthesia alone, local anesthesia with sedation (also called MAC or twilight sleep), regional anesthesia, or general anesthesia. (See chapter 2 for more information on anesthesia choices.) The type of anesthesia depends on the type of procedure you're having. For example, breast implants can be placed under MAC or general anesthesia; liposuction can be done under MAC; a facelift (rhytidectomy) can be done under MAC or general anesthesia; and nose reshaping (rhinoplasty) can be done under local anesthesia, MAC, or general anesthesia. An anesthesiologist is not present when a procedure is done with a topical anesthetic or only local anesthetic. In such circumstances, the surgeon may prescribe oral sedative medication to be taken before the surgery. Some cosmetic surgeons also administer mild intravenous (IV) sedation; in that case, a nurse should be present to monitor the patient.

Most cosmetic surgeons work with a regular group of anesthesiologists or with a particular anesthesiologist. An anesthesiologist is *required* in cases involving deep sedation or general anesthesia. To have multiple procedures (such as a tummy tuck and liposuction) done in the same session requires a longer use of anesthesia. The anesthesiologist should be familiar with the surgery and plan for continued care in the immediate recovery period. Make sure that you've discussed all of these issues with your surgeon and the anesthesiologist—before the scalpel.

Dr. Dhar Warns: Be Careful with the Creams!

Topical anesthetics, otherwise called "numbing creams," may be applied to the skin before laser or light-based treatments, chemical facial peels, micro-dermabrasion, and injectables to minimize pain. Some places even encourage application of topicals before waxing hair off parts of your body.

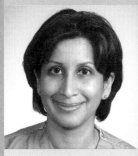

While topical anesthetics may seem risk-free, they should be used only with caution. First, the cream should be in a packaged, commercially labeled tube that is used *only for you*. And the U.S. Food and Drug Administration prohibits "compounded topical anesthetics" (mixing of the medication with other substances). The active ingredient in a topical cream or gel is a local anesthetic.

The most important factors are the amount of topical anesthetic used and the skin surface area to which it is applied. There have been deaths reported from topical overdose—rare, but it has happened. Topical anesthetics absorb slowly through the skin. They may enter the bloodstream, resulting in toxic reactions. Symptoms may include light-headedness, irregular heartbeat, and seizures. Severe allergic reactions can also occur. A large quantity of topical anesthetic should not be self-applied or applied without a medical professional monitoring you.

Unexpected Things Can Happen

As you prepare for the big day, it's important to learn about any potential surgical and anesthetic complications that may occur with your particular procedure(s) and your underlying health.

Complications during surgery, additional unplanned procedures, and prolonged duration of surgery are possibilities that the anesthesiologist has to be prepared to handle. For example, receiving an antibiotic can result in an allergic reaction severe enough to become a life-threatening medical emergency.

The overall rate of unexpected hospital admissions from a surgical center should be less than 2 percent. Before you choose a venue for your procedure, do your research! Some sites have better track records than others.

Unplanned admissions for overnight or a longer hospital stay are an unwelcome event for doctors, patient care providers, and, of course, the patients themselves. It's important to make sure the anesthesiologist has the equipment and back-up assistance to handle any situation—both routine and unexpected. If you choose to have the procedure in a non-hospital setting, a hospital should be nearby to transfer you quickly via ambulance in case of an emergency.

Facts to find out before the surgery:

- Is the procedure commonly performed at that location?
- In case of an emergency, what provisions are available?
- Which hospital will you be taken to, if necessary, and how far away is it?
- Does the surgeon have admitting privileges at the hospital?

Aim for a Quick Recovery

Recovery room issues such as nausea, vomiting, pain, bleeding, and wound drainage are just as real in a cosmetic procedure as in any other surgical procedure, so don't assume that outpatient procedures don't require follow-up care. If the surgery is done in an ambulatory surgery center, expect a next-day follow-up phone call from the facility or anesthesiologist to check that you are recovering properly at home. Make sure you have a contact number for the anesthesiologist on hand, just in case you need to call hours or days later.

Your speedy return to daily life and feeling happier are hallmarks of success for you, your surgeon, and your anesthesiologist. Facts to find out:

- Where will you recover immediately after the procedure?
- Does the facility have a recovery area?
- Who will monitor you in the recovery area? The surgeon, a nurse, or the anesthesiologist?
- What is the post-operative follow-up plan by the anesthesiologist?
- Are you expected to go home right after the procedure?

Adios! Anesthesia Abroad

The rising cost of health care in the United States has led to the phenomenon of "medical tourism." An increasing number of Americans are traveling to other countries for dental work, surgery, and other medical care. Thailand, Costa Rica, Mexico, Argentina, and several countries in Europe are favorite destinations for those wanting procedures at much lower prices.

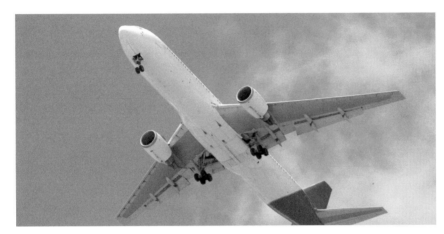

ON YOUR WAY ABROAD

Not surprisingly, most medical tourists seek cosmetic surgery. The financial savings can be enormous.

If this option tempts you, be sure to ask many, *many* questions before scheduling a procedure abroad. This will help you to avoid bad outcomes. Do your homework. Go online and "chat" with other medical tourists. Learn from their experiences. Find out everything you can about the procedure, the surgeon, the hospital or other location, and the after-care. And don't forget to learn about the anesthesia. Another country may follow standards for anesthetic care, sterilization techniques, facility certifications, physician qualification, and medical products that differ from U.S. standards. It also may be harder for you to establish a relationship with the surgeon and anesthesiologist in the other country.

It's a good thing to save money. But you also want to be sure you are safe and get beautiful results from whatever venue you choose for your procedure.

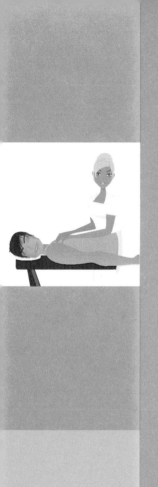

A Day at the Medi-spa

A new service called a **medi-spa** has become popular in the world of cosmetic medicine. A medi-spa may be a doctor's luxurious office enhanced with a support staff of aestheticians (people who are trained to care for your skin), nutritionists, and beauty consultants. Some medi-spas are found in non-traditional locations, such as shopping malls and beauty salons.

Medi-spas mainly offer non-surgical procedures such as facials, laser treatments, and pharmaceutical injectables (for example, Botox and Restylane). Anesthesia—if needed—for these types of treatments is limited to local or topical anesthetics. (Read this chapter's Panch-Line to learn about topicals.) Other non-surgical treatments such as aromatherapy, massage therapy, reflexology, nutrition counseling, grooming, and beauty tips make the destination a true spa.

It may be tempting to go to such facilities for a lower-priced Botox injection—but keep in mind that the price of Botox from the manufacturer, Allergan, is always the same. A lower-priced treatment may not be the genuine product, or it may be very diluted, and the person who delivers the treatment may not be well qualified. Thus, your results may not be as great as you had anticipated.

The regulation of medi-spas outside of a physician's office varies from state to state. There are no national standards for medi-spas, no oversight organizations—there isn't even a recognized definition of what a medi-spa is. A number of medi-spa facilities are owned by corporations and are staffed by persons with little or no training in dealing with medical complications and emergencies. Sometimes a medical doctor may have signed on as the "director," but he may not be physically present to supervise treatments.

Your safety is ensured when a physician who is board-certified in cosmetic procedures (a dermatologist or plastic surgeon) is available on-site at the time of laser and light-based treatments or injectables. A reputable location that offers physician-supervised treatments is a satisfying experience.

Prescriptives: Be a Better Consumer

☐ Before you decide on cosmetic surgery, get to know the credentials and experience of the surgeon and anesthesiologist who will be taking care of you.

_____

_____

☐ Make sure the person who is advertised as doing the cosmetic surgery is the one who will actually perform your procedure. After all, you are paying for your dreams!

_____

_____

☐ Get a complete medical check-up before you have cosmetic surgery. This is to make sure other health problems don't interfere with the anesthesia and your recovery. _____

_____

☐ Find out the anesthetic plan before your surgery. Remember, if you are having multiple procedures done in one session, you will be under anesthesia longer.

_____

_____

☐ Consider taking some time off from work after major cosmetic surgery. This will help you adjust to the new you. _____

_____

CHAPTERNINE

weighty matters:
what about
the heavy patient?

Obesity has become a global and particularly
an American concern. The latest data from the National Center for Health Statistics show that nearly one-third of U.S. adults ages twenty and older—that is, more than sixty million adults—are overweight or obese. The weight problem is not just limited to adults. About twenty-five million children and adolescents in the United States are overweight or nearly overweight. Increased weight in a child leads to a higher risk of obesity as an adult.

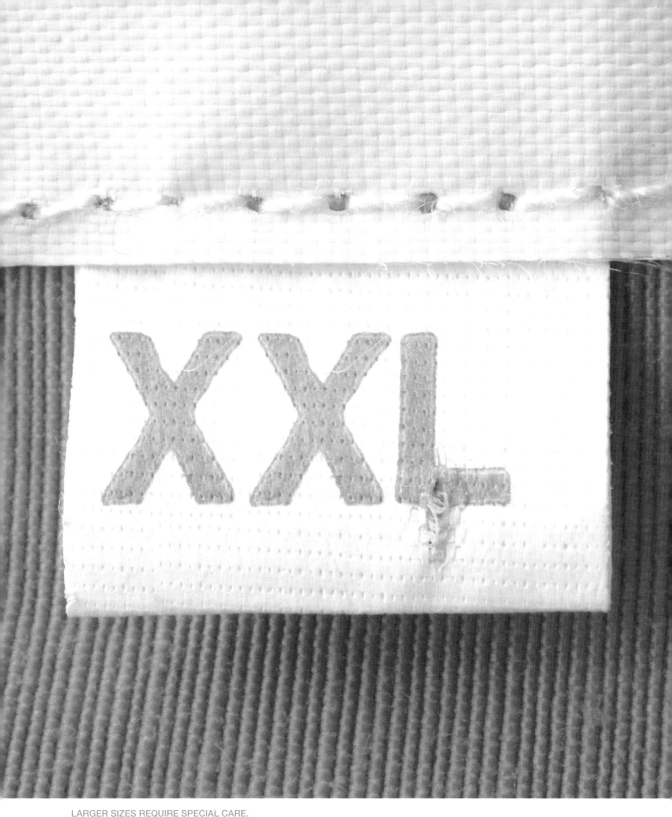

LARGER SIZES REQUIRE SPECIAL CARE.

Do You Measure Up?

What officially labels a person as being overweight or obese? Health professionals and epidemiologists use a weight-to-height ratio called the **body mass index** (BMI) to estimate body fat. BMI can be calculated by dividing a person's weight in kilograms (1 kilogram = 2.2 pounds) by the square of his height in meters (1 meter = 3.3 feet). That is:

$$\text{body mass index (BMI)} = \text{kilogram/meter}^2$$

- A BMI under 18.5 is considered underweight.
- A BMI of 18.5 to 24.9 is considered normal weight.
- A BMI of 25.0 to 29.9 is considered overweight.
- A BMI of 30.0 to 39.9 is considered obese.
- A BMI of 40.0 or higher is considered morbidly obese.

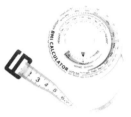

BODY MASS INDEX (BMI) TABLE

BMI	19	20	21	22	23	24	25	26	27	28	29	30	31	32	33	34	35
height								weight (in pounds)									
4'10" (58")	91	96	100	105	110	115	119	124	129	134	138	143	148	153	158	162	167
4'11" (59")	94	99	104	109	114	119	124	128	133	138	143	148	153	158	163	168	173
5' (60")	97	102	107	112	118	123	128	133	138	143	148	153	158	163	168	174	179
5'1" (61")	100	106	111	116	122	127	132	137	143	148	153	158	164	169	174	180	185
5'2" (62")	104	109	115	120	126	131	136	142	147	153	158	164	169	175	180	186	191
5'3" (63")	107	113	118	124	130	135	141	146	152	158	163	169	175	180	186	191	197
5'4" (64")	110	116	122	128	134	140	145	151	157	163	169	174	180	186	192	197	204
5'5" (65")	114	120	126	132	138	144	150	156	162	168	174	180	186	192	198	204	210
5'6" (66")	118	124	130	136	142	148	155	161	167	173	179	186	192	198	204	210	216
5'7" (67")	121	127	134	140	146	153	159	166	172	178	185	191	198	204	211	217	223
5'8" (68")	125	131	138	144	151	158	164	171	177	184	190	197	203	210	216	223	230
5'9" (69")	128	135	142	149	155	162	169	176	182	189	196	203	209	216	223	230	236
5'10" (70")	132	139	146	153	160	167	174	181	188	195	202	209	216	222	229	236	243
5'11" (71")	136	143	150	157	165	172	179	186	193	200	208	215	222	229	236	243	250
6' (72")	140	147	154	162	169	177	184	191	199	206	213	221	228	235	242	250	258
6'1" (73")	144	151	159	166	174	182	189	197	204	212	219	227	235	242	250	257	265
6'2" (74")	148	155	163	171	179	186	194	202	210	218	225	233	241	249	256	264	272
6'3" (75")	152	160	168	176	184	192	200	208	216	224	232	240	248	256	264	272	279

Source: Evidence Report of Clinical Guidelines on the Identification, Evaluation, and Treatment of Overweight and Obesity in Adults, 1998. NIH/National Heart, Lung, and Blood Institute (NHLBI)

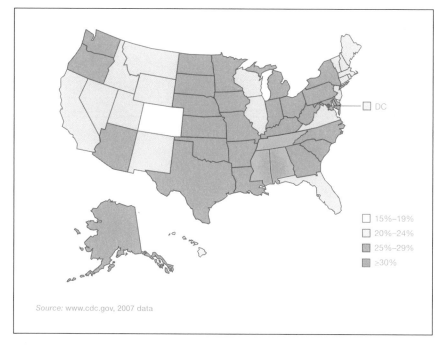

□	15%–19%
□	20%–24%
▨	25%–29%
■	≥30%

Source: www.cdc.gov, 2007 data

THE PREVALENCE OF OBESITY (BMI≥30) AMONG U.S. ADULTS, 2007

The Overweight Patient and Anesthesia

The increasing weight of the population has challenged anesthesiologists to modify their practices and techniques. Overweight or obese patients can receive all types of anesthetics—local, monitored anesthesia care (MAC), regional, and general. But some extra factors have to be kept in mind by both the doctor and the patient.

A patient's weight is a major factor in anesthetic care. If you are overweight, it is essential that you tell the anesthesiologist about any co-existing health issues. Patients who are heavy are more likely to have heart disease, high blood pressure, stroke, type 2 diabetes, gastro-esophageal reflux disease (GERD), difficulty breathing, and sleep apnea. Even young people are more likely to experience heart failure and blockage in their heart vessels if they're overweight.

Such health issues mean that precautions need to be taken, from the pre-operative evaluation to post-operative recovery. Anesthesiologists have begun to use new and innovative ways to handle larger patients.

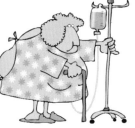

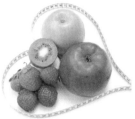

⚠️ *Increased patient weight presents special challenges for anesthesiologists. Let your anesthesia provider know if you have gained a large amount of weight since your last surgery. What was routine for you as a slim person may not be routine if you have gained a significant amount of weight since your previous surgery.*

Here are some examples of what affects anesthetic care for people who are overweight or obese. Keep in mind these issues are not applicable to all heavy persons.

Positioning on the Operating Table

A larger operating table and extra padding may be needed to properly position the obese patient in the operating room. Extra pillows may be used to prop up the head, as lying flat on the table may be uncomfortable due to excess weight of the abdomen and chest.

Access to Veins

The anesthetic process begins with a good working intravenous (IV) line. But finding good veins on an overweight patient may take extra time and effort. Sometimes an arterial line or central venous line may need to be placed to achieve reliable blood pressure readings and venous access.

A blood pressure cuff may be placed on the forearm or leg if the upper arm is too large for the cuff to go around.

Breathing Changes

The resting blood oxygen level may be lower and the carbon dioxide level may be higher in obese patients with sleep apnea. It is part of the obesity hypoventilation syndrome or Pickwickian syndrome (named after the robust character in Charles Dickens' novel *Pickwick Papers*). Anesthesiologists have to be extra-cautious of this situation, because even a slight decline in the breathing rate from a small amount of sedative means a faster drop in oxygen levels. IV sedation becomes a delicate balance between keeping the patient comfortable and maintaining acceptable blood oxygen levels.

Aspiration Precautions

Even though all patients are required to follow fasting guidelines, an overweight person's stomach may empty slower than normal. This creates a higher chance of aspiration—when inhaled stomach contents enter the lungs—because the stomach may still be full even though many hours have passed since the person last ate a meal.

But don't be nervous. Anesthesiologists use a maneuver to prevent aspiration. Quick insertion of the breathing tube at the start of general anesthesia blocks the chance of stomach contents coming back up and entering the lungs.

Intubation Difficulties

If a general anesthetic is required, the anesthesiologist may take extra precautions when placing a breathing tube (intubating) in the obese patient's windpipe (trachea). A larger neck and more fat under the chin may increase the technical difficulty of intubation and ventilation. Today, anesthesiologists use specially designed devices (GlideScope, Fastrach, Airtraq) that make placement of the endotracheal tube quick and easy.

On some occasions the anesthesiologist may decide it is safer to place the tube before starting a general anesthetic. That means while the patient is awake. To do this, the patient's mouth and throat are first numbed with a local anesthetic so that tube insertion is not uncomfortable. Some mild sedation is given to minimize anxiety. A flexible **fiberoptic bronchoscope** (camera) may be used to guide the breathing tube into proper position. The idea behind this technique is that if a person is kept breathing, his oxygen level won't drop. The patient is made unconscious immediately after the tube placement is confirmed.

The anesthesiologist can place an endotracheal tube while maintaining the patient's comfort and minimizing his anxiety. General anesthesia is started immediately after the tube placement is confirmed.

Regional Anesthesia Challenges

Regional anesthesia is often used in overweight patients to reduce the risks related to airway control and diminished breathing from sedatives. Techniques such as spinal, epidural, and peripheral nerve blocks are

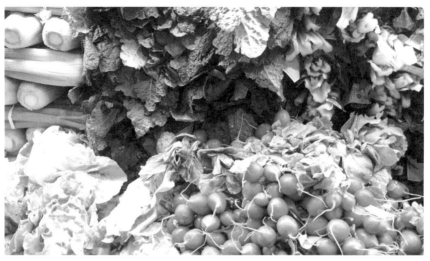

THINK HEALTHY.

done routinely and safely on thousands of overweight patients each day, but they still demand expert skill. It can be a challenge for the anesthesiologist to find the usual anatomic "landmarks" on an overweight patient.

Recently, the use of ultrasound technology has made providing regional anesthesia easier by allowing anesthesiologists to actually see the nerves to be blocked. Used alone or with a light general anesthetic, regional anesthesia lessens the effect on the patient's respiratory system. It also helps with post-operative pain control.

Medication Modification

The anesthetic dosage and requirements for people who are overweight are altered by changes in absorption, metabolism, and clearance of medication. An obese patient may need more or less of a certain medication to achieve the same effect as in slim patients. Over the past few years, new anesthetic drugs with fast onset, short duration of action, and fewer side effects have been introduced.

On to the Recovery Room

When a surgery or other procedure is finished, the anesthesiologist's job is not over. In the recovery room, the overweight patient may experience a drop in oxygen levels because of the lingering effects of anesthetic agents such as opioids. Additional oxygen may have to be given at this time. The anesthesiologist continues to watch for this and any other possible complications.

Depending on the type of surgery and the clinical condition of the patient, **mechanical ventilation** may need to be continued. The endotracheal tube is removed only when the doctors are sure that the patient is stable and strong enough to breathe on his own.

Anesthesiologists Are Standing By!

Every day, anesthesia providers are expanding their knowledge of the special care needed for our "growing" population. You can feel confident that they are better prepared for the unique challenges involved in treating people of all shapes and sizes.

 Prescriptives: Be a Better Consumer

☐ Look up your body mass index (BMI) before having a medical procedure done.

_____

☐ Let your anesthesiologist know if you have gained a substantial amount of weight since your last medical procedure. _____

_____

☐ If you are overweight, let your doctors know about any health problems that you may have, such as high blood pressure, diabetes, or heartburn. _____

_____

☐ Talk with your doctor about whether it's possible for you to diet or exercise before the surgery. Following a healthy diet and getting regular exercise put you in more control of your life. _____

_____

☐ Let your doctors know if you currently smoke or formerly smoked cigarettes.

_____

CHAPTERTEN

labor of love:
enjoy childbirth

Should women have a right to choose a pain-free
delivery of a baby through the use of anesthesia?
Or should they go the natural route and use absolutely
no medication, no matter how much they might suffer
while giving birth?

Thankfully, women can make the decision for themselves these days. And anesthesiologists are well prepared to meet their individual needs—and to respect
each woman's wishes.

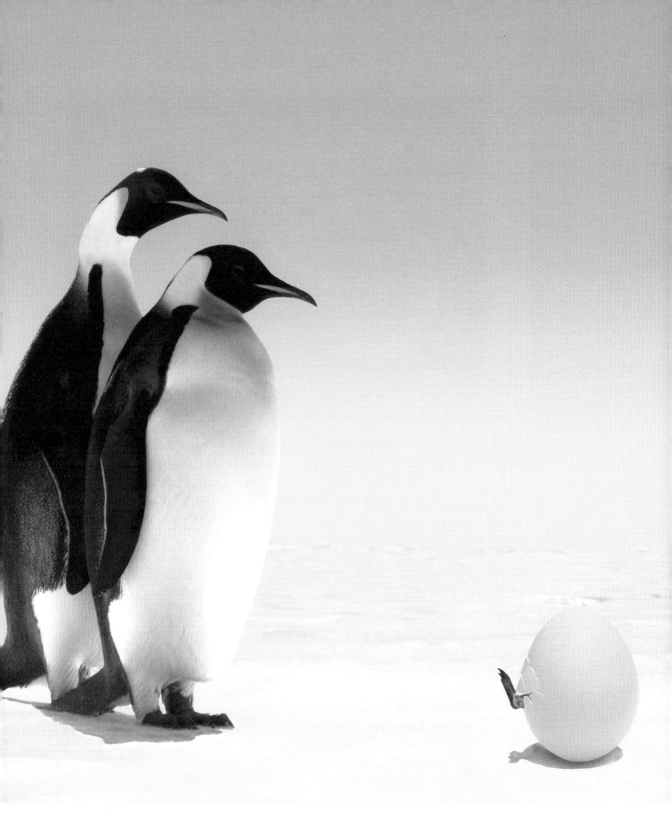

CHILDBIRTH IS AN IMPORTANT EVENT IN ALL SOCIETIES.

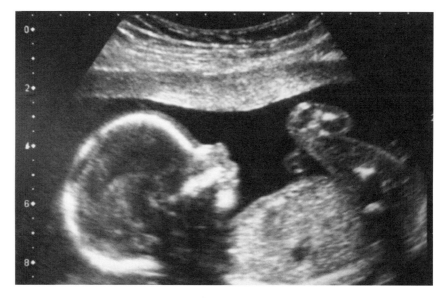

A FETUS IN THE WOMB

Life in the Labor Ward

Obstetric anesthesia has a special place in the world of medicine. This specialty demands quick thinking, technical ability, and physical stamina. Obstetric anesthesiologists have a great deal of responsibility. They work closely with obstetricians (doctors who see women through the pregnancy and delivery process) to make sure that both mother and baby are safe and happy.

The busier the **labor suite** (the area where women go through the birth process), the greater the number of anesthesia providers needed. That's why larger medical centers typically staff the labor ward with a full A Team (team of anesthesia providers) to make sure that all situations—regular deliveries and emergencies—can be covered around the clock.

Things change fast in a labor suite. The place can be quiet one minute, and a hive of activity the very next.

A patient can be sitting quietly in bed with her epidural (see the discussion in chapter 2 on the types of anesthetics) in place one minute—and the next minute a change in the fetal heart rate could mean she will be raced to the operating room for an emergency **cesarean section** (C-section).

Meanwhile, another patient on the brink of delivery may ask for an epidural despite her initial decision to give birth "naturally" without medication.

A few minutes later three more women in various stages of labor could be requesting epidurals.

Soon after, an obstetrician could decide to do a C-section on another patient who has been laboring for hours without making much progress.

And don't forget the special demands on the medical staff for women carrying twins, triplets, or breech babies!

PanchLines

Dr. Dhar Reports: How Common Is the Use of Anesthesia in Labor and Delivery?

In the United States, epidural anesthesia plays a major role in the birthing process. Each year about one million pregnant women choose to have epidural anesthesia during labor. Over 50 percent of women giving birth at hospitals use epidural anesthesia.

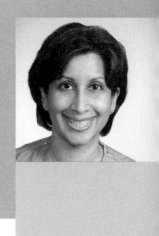

The Pregnant Woman Is Different

You'll hardly be surprised to learn that there are differences between pregnant and non-pregnant women—and it's not just about the obvious, growing "bump"!

For one thing, medical professionals have two patients to care for—the woman and her unborn child.

For another, every system in the body changes during pregnancy. The woman's body "mechanics" change. She will use more oxygen and have a larger blood volume and increased heart rate. Her blood pressure will be slightly lower, her stomach will empty more slowly. She will also have weight gain and a greater sensitivity of the brain to anesthetics. These are just some of the important factors that her doctors must bear in mind.

Enjoy Labor? You Must Be Kidding!

Regional anesthesia is the preferred technique for a patient in labor. Epidural or combined spinal-epidural (CSE) anesthetics are done on millions of women every year throughout the world. Both of these are regional anesthetics that allow women to have a safe and *comfortable* birthing experience. Women can see and hold their baby immediately after delivery.

Pain control for labor can be carried out by intravenous (IV) medication or regional techniques. (See chapter 7 for a full discussion on pain management.) Early labor pain can be relieved with pain medication such as meperidine (Demerol). But as labor progresses and the pain increases in intensity, IV medications may not be enough.

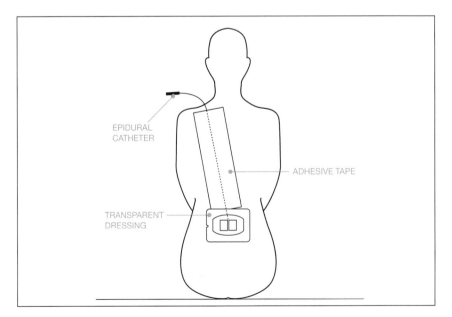

AN EPIDURAL TAPED UP ALONG THE BACK

In the later stages, the intense pain is better controlled with epidural medication.

The anesthesiologist places an epidural or CSE upon the woman's request. (The woman's labor partner is asked to step out of the room at this time.) A nurse remains in the room to help position the patient. The epidural is used for the entire duration of labor through vaginal delivery. The epidural catheter can be connected to a patient-controlled analgesia (PCA) device, and a mild dose of local anesthetic and opioid is given through the epidural catheter by a pump. The **walking epidural** provides pain relief while still allowing the woman to move around a bit.

If a C-section is required, a stronger dose of local anesthetic is given through the existing epidural catheter, so the patient is numbed and cannot move from the chest downward. After the delivery, the epidural catheter can be promptly removed. Some institutions continue to use the catheter after surgery with **patient-controlled epidural analgesia (PCEA).** Spinal anesthesia can also be used for a planned or, if time permits, emergency C-section.

FRESHLY HATCHED

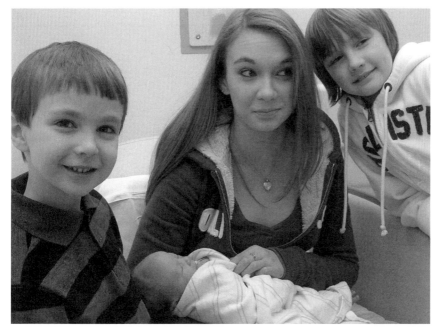

THE BABY'S BIG SISTER AND BROTHERS WELCOME THE NEW ARRIVAL.

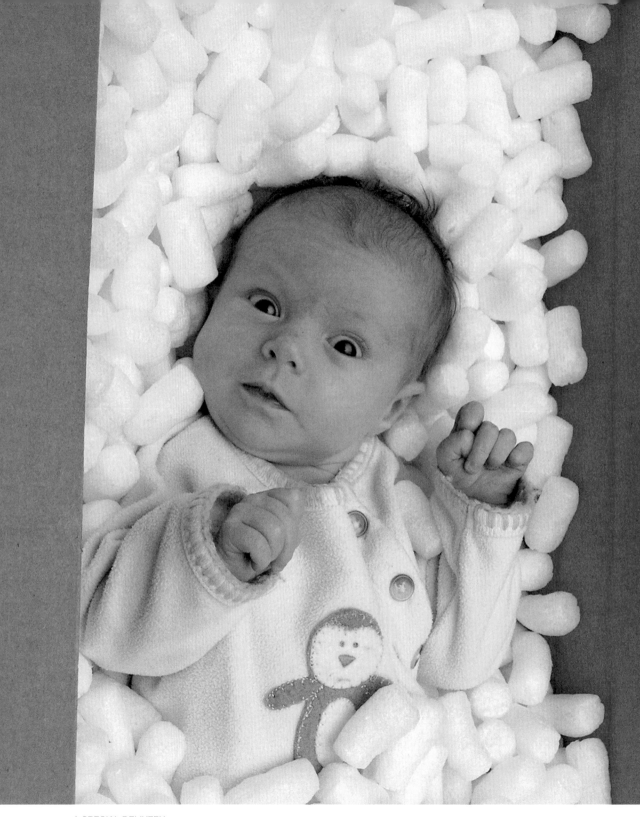

A SPECIAL DELIVERY

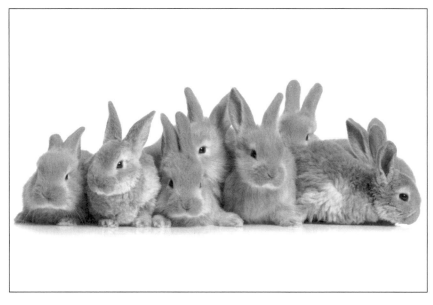

FERTILITY!

Safety First

General anesthesia is used for C-sections when regional anesthesia is refused by the patient, is best avoided (for example, because of risk of bleeding or extensive back surgery), is difficult to place, or does not work effectively. It can also be given when emergency conditions prevent placement of a regional anesthetic.

⚠ *One of the most important changes during pregnancy is in a woman's airway anatomy. From an anesthesiologist's standpoint, the pregnant woman is more likely to be a "difficult intubation" (see the section on airway management in chapter 2) than a non-pregnant female. This means there is a greater chance that the anesthesiologist may not be able to see the woman's vocal cords. Then it becomes a challenge to quickly insert a breathing tube (endotracheal tube) into the windpipe (trachea) after general anesthetic drugs are given. Despite this vital concern, you can rest assured that general anesthesia is performed safely every day on obstetric patients with the careful planning and expertise of anesthesiologists.*

Surgical Delivery

The cesarean section rate has increased dramatically in the United States. In 1970, only 5 percent of births were by C-section. The C-section rate in the United States today is nearly 40 percent, especially in urban hospitals. This may be due to the following reasons:

- Improvements in fetal monitoring encourage delivery at the first sign of fetal distress.
- Advances in reproductive technology have increased the incidence of multiple births that require surgical interventions.
- More women over age forty are giving birth for the first time.
- Pregnant women may choose C-section to avoid labor entirely.
- Legal liability concerns often create an environment of caution.

A C-section can be done under regional anesthesia (spinal, epidural, or combined techniques) or general anesthesia. Many women are concerned about whether regional anesthesia prolongs labor. An important study published by the *New England Journal of Medicine* in 2005 noted that CSE placement early in labor did not increase the rate of C-section delivery. The CSE provided better pain control and a shorter duration of labor than IV medication.

A CESAREAN BIRTH

A Comforting Range of Options

Anesthesia today can be part of a positive birthing experience. Thanks to medical advances, labor can be a comfortable and exciting experience for both mother and family.

 Prescriptives: Be a Better Consumer

☐ **Keep a log of how you feel your body is changing during pregnancy. This includes weight gain, ease of breathing, and the appearance of back pain.**

_____
_____

☐ **Ask your obstetrician about your labor pain management options.** _____

_____

☐ If you are planning to have an epidural placed during labor, ask to meet your anesthesiologist when you enter the labor ward. This way you can ask questions and discuss the procedure. _____

_____

☐ You may consider natural childbirth (without anesthesia) as an option. This depends on your level of pain tolerance, your health issues, issues during your pregnancy, and obstetrician's practice style. _____

_____

☐ Surround yourself with things that will help your emotional needs during labor— an iPod with your favorite music, interesting magazines, or a favorite pillow.

_____

_____

CHAPTERELEVEN

the smallest breaths:
when your child needs anesthesia

In the past half century, rapid advances in anesthesia have vastly improved the care of even the youngest of patients. Anesthesia for the young is extremely safe today, thanks to modern technology, new drugs, and a better understanding of pain management. Some anesthesiologists specialize in pediatrics—the branch of medicine concerned with the treatment of infants and children. (There are also pediatric surgeons, doctors who operate solely on infants and children.)

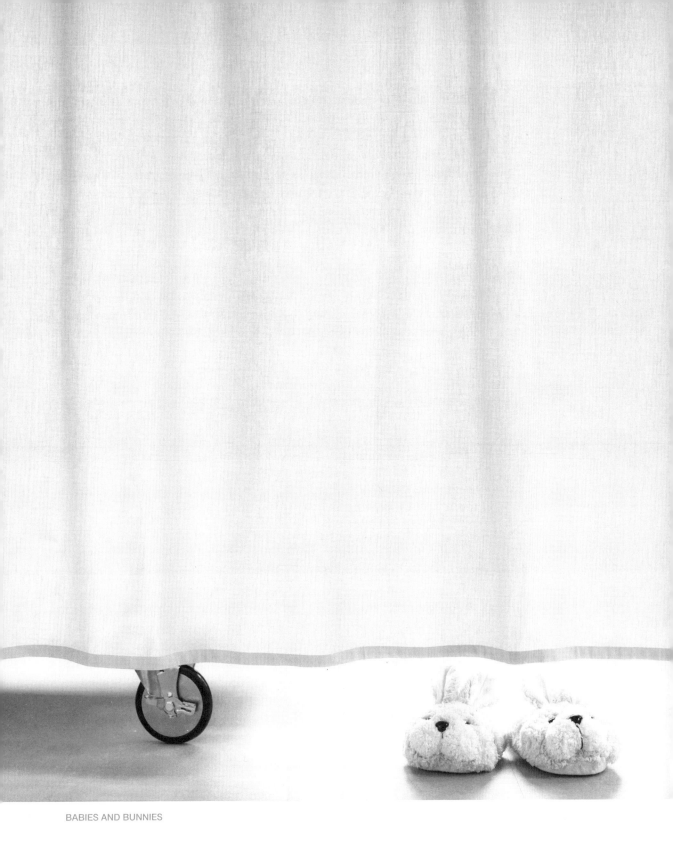

The field of **pediatric anesthesia** has evolved separately, because there are important differences in the physical characteristics of infants and small children as compared to adults. Technology and research are helping **pediatric anesthesiologists** to care for smaller and smaller **premies**—pre-term infants (those born before thirty-seven weeks of pregnancy). These doctors have the skills to care for not only healthy children but also those with congenital (existing at birth) defects and serious health issues that occur after birth.

It's Not Just the Size

Young people are not simply "little adults." Compared to adults, children have major physical and developmental differences that change over months and years. Because of this, anesthesiologists divide children by age, which helps in choosing anesthesia equipment, monitoring, and drug dosing.

Age Divisions

Neonate (newborn): birth to 4 weeks of age
Infant: 1 month to 1 year
Toddler: 1 to 3 years
Child: 3 to 12 years
Teenager: 13 to 18 years

Anesthesiologists use different techniques in airway management (see chapter 2), temperature control, and fluid and blood measurements when caring for **neonates** (newborns), infants, and small children. For example, the heart rate and breathing pattern of a neonate are faster than in a five-year-old child. Intubation of the premature infant and newborn is more challenging than in adults because of physical differences. Oxygen levels in newborns, premature infants, and children drop rapidly after starting anesthesia because their bodies use oxygen faster. This calls for expertise in managing the pediatric airway.

The precise dosing of medication in children is based on their weight. Drugs must be dosed carefully, because the effects can last longer and be more intense.

What would be considered a small amount of blood loss in an adult is a massive blood loss for a newborn. That's why the anesthesiologist must pay careful attention to blood and other fluid measurements. Factors to consider during a procedure are the extent of surgery, daily fluid needs, urine output, and blood loss to maintain the patient's stability. This may involve weighing sponges to accurately measure blood loss!

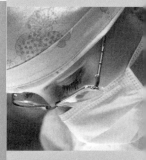

Not-So-Small Differences!

Here are just some of the physical differences between children and adults:

- Newborns are nose breathers by nature.
- Neonates utilize oxygen two to three times faster than adults.
- The lungs in a newborn mature to adult characteristics by eight to ten years of age.
- Newborns, infants, and children up to age five years have higher breathing rates than adults. The rates approach adult values (twelve to twenty breaths per minute) by the teenage years.
- Newborns, infants, and children have higher heart rates.
- The blood circulation rate in newborns is two to three times that of adults.
- Newborns, infants, and young children have lower blood pressure. Blood pressure reaches adult values by about five years of age.
- The kidney's capacity to clear drugs from the body is diminished in infants.
- The body composition of newborns and infants contains a greater amount of water.
- The blood of a newborn has a different biological structure and oxygen-carrying mechanics. It is gradually replaced, over months, with adult red blood cells.
- In infants, the liver is slower to clear medications. This means that the effects of drugs can last longer.
- Newborns have less sugar (glucose) stores in their body. This makes them more prone to low blood sugar levels.

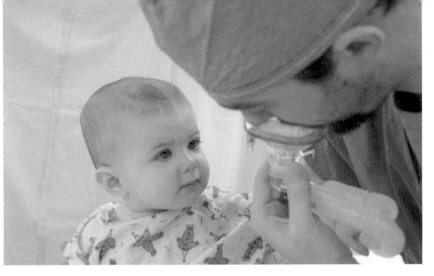

DEMONSTRATING A FACE MASK

Preparing for the Big Day

Your child needs surgery. You're frightened and unsure about what will happen. Your experience with anesthesia won't be the same as your child's. So how can you lessen your fear and anxiety?

First, gather information about the anesthesia planned for your child. If possible, speak to a member of the anesthesia team before the procedure—this is a great way to learn about the surgery *and* the anesthesia. The hospital's anesthesia department may offer information by phone, in booklets, or even in a video.

Before meeting the anesthesiologist, write down any questions and concerns you and your child have. This is an opportunity to take an active role in the anesthetic care. For instance, will you be able to accompany the child into the operating room? What type of anesthesia will she be given? Will your child have an intravenous (IV) line when she leaves surgery? How long will she be in the recovery room? When will she be able to see you?

The anesthesiologist first gathers information about the child and then gives a brief physical examination. The information collected includes:

- Issues during pregnancy
- Medical issues immediately after birth
- Birth weight and age (how many weeks from conception to birth)
- Apgar scores (measure skin color, heart rate, reflexes, muscle tone, and breathing)

- Length of hospital stay after birth
- Hospitalizations or emergency room visits
- Current health problems
- Allergies
- Results of previous anesthesia experiences, if any
- Current medications
- Emotional needs

Blood tests are usually ordered only if there is a particular problem (for example, sickle-cell disease) or a major operation like heart surgery is being done. They are not always ordered for routine operations, such as placing ear tubes or a tonsillectomy.

Calming Words

You'll need to tell your child about the procedure in an age-appropriate way. Reassurance that you will be close by is the most helpful.

Describing the process beforehand helps ease a youngster's fears. Use simple terms and examples to prepare for the operating room experience. For instance, you might say: "A light will be attached to your finger. A fruit-flavored mask may be placed over your nose and mouth to breathe into."

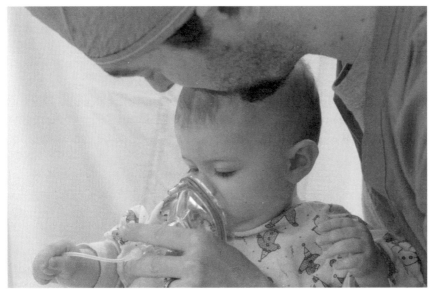

TRYING ON THE FACE MASK

Feeding and Fasting

Nowadays, prolonged fasting before surgery is not recommended for children. Abstaining from eating and drinking causes fluid loss, low blood sugar, and irritability. Allowing the young patient to have clear fluids up to two hours before the surgery helps provide a smoother start. Some medical centers may allow a child to have a small, soft breakfast if the procedure is scheduled for the afternoon.

Anesthetics for the Young

Many anesthetic techniques and medications are available for youngsters. Some of the same anesthetic drugs used in adults are modified for children, but doses are downsized based on weight. Depending on the circumstance and policy of the medical center, sedatives may be given before a child enters the operating room. These drugs are given to lessen fear and anxiety, ease separation from parents, help cooperation during the start of anesthesia, and prevent children from remembering what happens after leaving their parents. Infants under one year don't understand what is happening, so such medications are not needed.

General anesthesia is the most common technique used in infants and children. It is helpful for a child to be in physical contact with someone during the start of general anesthesia. If an intravenous line can be placed with finesse, anesthetic medications can be given through it. In some centers, the parent or guardian is permitted to enter the operating room and hold a child in their lap as the clear plastic anesthetic mask is placed. The anesthetic begins when the child is asked to breathe a mixture of enriched oxygen and anesthetic gas. A gas such as sevoflurane is pleasant smelling (non-pungent) and works very quickly, so the child is unconscious in less than a minute.

An IV line to administer the rest of the medications is placed after the child is asleep. Other interventions such as intubation and additional monitors (such as an arterial line) are placed after a child is fully anesthetized. At the end of the surgery, the anesthetic gas is turned off, and the child emerges from anesthesia quickly.

Regional anesthesia such as spinal, epidural, and local nerve blocks are also used in the pediatric setting. Of course, parental consent is re-

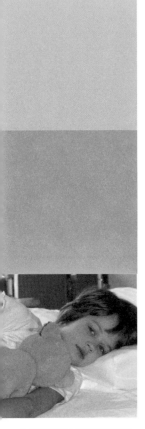

A FAVORITE TOY CAN BE COMFORTING.

quired, and not every child is a candidate. Because of significant physical differences between adults and children, regional anesthesia equipment is modified to smaller sizes, and drug doses are downsized as well.

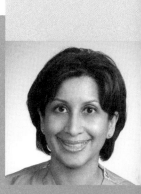

Waking Up and Getting About

After surgery, your child will be transferred to the recovery room or, if required, the intensive care unit. Nurses and doctors make sure the child is stable before you are permitted to visit the bedside.

In the recovery room, a child's vital signs and pain level are regularly monitored, just as they would be in an adult. Some children need to be taken directly from the operating room to the intensive care unit for further care.

It is not uncommon for children to wake up from anesthesia feeling disoriented, confused, and unsure of where they are. At such times, seeing a familiar face, hearing a comforting voice, and being held by a family member is the best medicine. Comfort and reassurance from family at the bedside can help curb the need to give sedative medication.

If a child is still upset even after being comforted by a loved one, the anesthesiologist considers the need for pain medication or sedation.

Children and even pre-term infants experience pain to the same degree as adults. Pain management has been extended to the care of even the tiniest babies. Medications such as morphine and rectal Tylenol can be given to infants and children for pain control. (See the general discussion of pain management in chapter 7.)

Although many children may leave the hospital on the same day as the surgery, some children are not eligible for such ambulatory procedures. This group includes pre-term infants and infants with a history of breathing problems, heart problems, and metabolic problems.

More Children Are Yet to Come!

- The United States, at a population of 300 million, is the world's third most-populous country, after China and India, and has the highest population growth rate of all industrialized countries.
- The U.S. population is set to reach 400 million by 2039.

Source: www.prb.org (Population Reference Bureau), 2008 data

Small Breaths Count

There are times when a child needs to have a routine health checkup and times when the need for a medical intervention or surgery arises . . . unexpectedly. Pediatric anesthesiologists have the know-how for getting a young one through a simple hernia operation or corrective heart surgery. Nowadays children can undergo as many types of surgeries and procedures as their adult counterparts. Rapid advances in pediatric medicine and surgery have been an impetus for evolving the anesthetic care of young ones. As the population in the world grows through better health care and greater life expectancy, so will the number of children who survive with complex medical needs. The population under the age

of eighteen is expected to increase by 20 percent over the next fifteen years. Likewise, the demand for health care for children will increase. Participating in your child's anesthetic experience will help even the youngest get through the toughest times.

Rx **Prescriptives:** Be a Better Consumer

 Keep a list of your child's medical history, including medications. _____

_____

 Meet with the anesthesiologist before your child is taken to the operating room. It is a great opportunity to ask questions. _____

_____

 Find out if any special monitors will be used during your child's surgery. _____

_____

 Find out when you will be able to join your child after surgery. _____

_____

 Ask how soon after the procedure your child will be able to go home. _____

_____

CHAPTERTWELVE {

smile!
dentistry
and oral surgery

The thought of going to the dentist makes a lot
of people nervous. You may be putting off getting a rot-
ten tooth pulled, because you can't stop thinking about
the giant needle meant to numb your gums. Even seeing the dentist's pick coming toward your mouth can
send a sharp tingle across your face. Sitting perfectly still
and holding your mouth open can test your nerves.

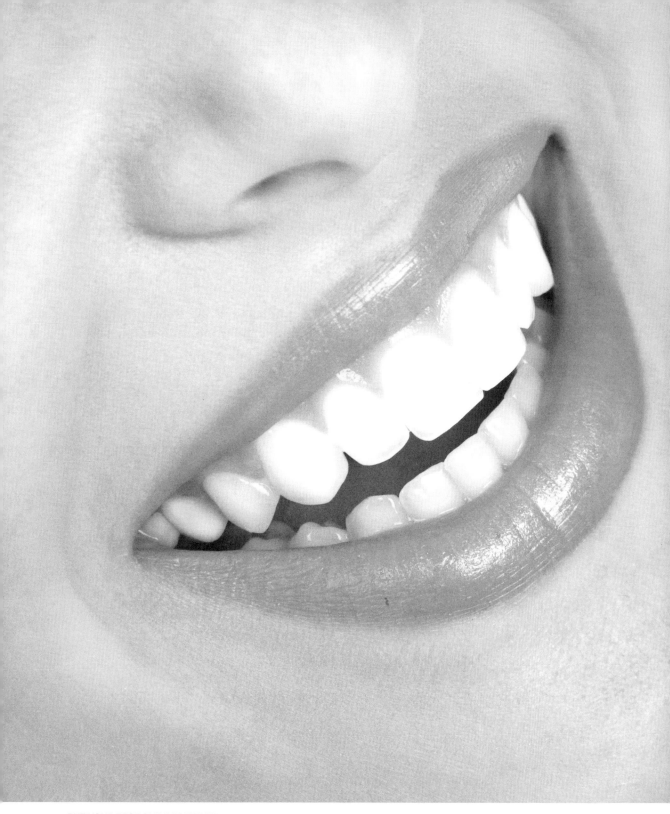

PUT YOUR BEST SMILE FORWARD.

Luckily, most dental procedures don't last long and are minimally invasive. Most people don't require anesthesia for a routine dental cleaning. But for tooth extraction and different types of dental surgery, it's the standard of care. Post-procedure pain can often be controlled with oral pain medications as simple as acetaminophen (Tylenol) or ibuprofen (Advil, Motrin).

Every day dentists treat patients who are scared and nervous. They also treat babies, children, and people with emotional and physical disabilities. Then there are those extensive surgical procedures when numbing the mouth is just the start.

Dentists Can Give Anesthesia?

Local anesthesia is the main method of pain control in dentistry, and all dentists are trained to give local anesthesia for office-based procedures. In addition, some dentists are trained in sedation and general anesthesia. That's because more than just an injection is needed for people who are very anxious or fidgety. The additional anesthesia helps the dentist perform a procedure more effectively on a patient who is not a moving target!

Dentists who use minimal sedation must complete formal training that meets with American Dental Association guidelines. Only those dentists who have completed an advanced education program accredited by the Commission on Dental Accreditation (CODA) are trained in deep sedation and general anesthesia, and are considered educationally qualified to use these in their practice.

Anytime anesthesia beyond a local injection is planned, a responsible adult companion needs to take you to the dental office before treatment begins. Your escort should accompany you home once you have fully recovered.

The Dentist's Arsenal for Your Comfort

Today dentists and oral surgeons have a wide array of drugs and techniques to help ease pain and anxiety. (See chapter 2 for a rundown on anesthetics and chapter 7 for a discussion on pain management.)

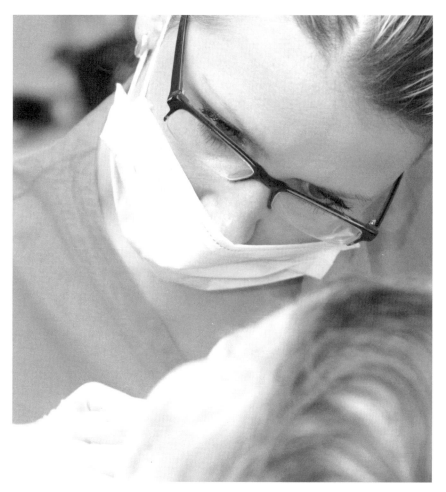

OPEN WIDE!

If a local anesthetic isn't enough, a twilight sleep with intravenous (IV) anesthetics or inhaling nitrous oxide ("laughing gas") can cloud your thoughts and calm you. And, if required, general anesthesia can render you totally unconscious.

⚠️ *It's very important that advanced anesthesia be limited only to patients who require it. Remember, anesthesia has risks, and not everyone is a candidate for general anesthesia. Anesthesia in a dental office should be taken as seriously as in a hospital. During the procedure, for example,*

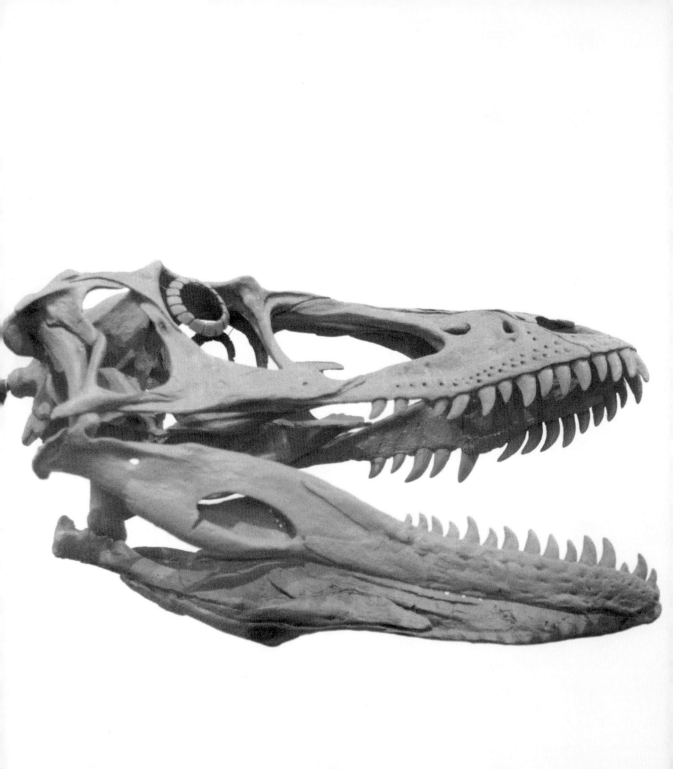

TEETH GET NOTICED!

*monitoring of heart rate and oxygen saturation is essential. As in any medical procedure, unexpected emergencies and complications can happen. The **dental/oral surgeon** has the knowledge and practical skills to treat emergencies, but a way to rapidly transfer a patient to a hospital must be available.*

On "Top" and Around

Topical anesthetics are applied with a swab to the surface of the gums and inside the mouth in order to ease or prevent pain. A dentist may use a topical anesthetic to numb the surface of the gums before injecting a strong local anesthetic. This is many people's first encounter with anesthesia.

The local anesthetic is injected around specific nerves to prevent pain in the gums, teeth, and mouth during treatment. All dentists have expertise in the application of local anesthetics, or what most people refer to as "novocaine." The local anesthetic usually outlasts the duration of the procedure so it often leaves you feeling like you have a "fat lip" and numbed tongue. Local anesthetics are commonly used in such procedures as filling cavities, preparing teeth for crowns, and treating gum disease.

PanchLines

Dr. Dhar Describes: Articaine—A New Local in the Neighborhood

Dentists may use a new local anesthetic called articaine (Septocaine) to numb the gums. It's stronger and acts faster than novocaine and lidocaine, and it's very safe. However, it should not be used to block specific nerves in the mouth, because there have been cases of long-term numbness reported after a lower jaw (mandibular) nerve block.

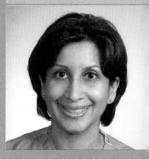

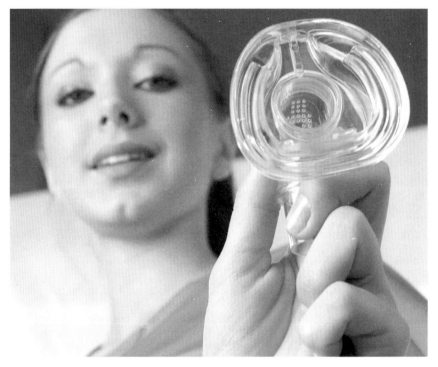

YOUR VIEW OF A FACE MASK

Taking the Edge Off

Sedative tablets, inhaled nitrous oxide/oxygen (laughing gas), and IV medications can be used with cooperative but anxious patients to help them relax during treatment. This twilight sleep, also called conscious sedation, can be given for tooth removal or short oral surgical procedures. It's also used in the care of young dental patients.

The oldest oral sedative used to relax adults before sitting in the dental chair is diazepam (Valium). Fast-onset and short-acting sedatives used for adults and children are triazolam (Halcion, Novodorm, Songar) and midazolam (Versed). Although triazolam is approved by the U.S. Food and Drug Administration for the short-term treatment of insomnia (having trouble sleeping), dentists like to use it because it provides effective and safe sedation for moderately anxious patients. A triazolam tablet can be swallowed (oral route) or placed under the tongue to dissolve (sublingual route) before an appointment. Midazolam is available in a syrup form. An additional dose of these drugs can be given in the dentist's office, or other medications such as inhaled nitrous oxide/oxygen can be added. Keep in mind that discharge from the office can be delayed due to prolonged sedation.

 There is a danger of slowed and shallow breathing if excessive doses of sedative drugs are given or if they are combined with a narcotic like fentanyl.

Sometimes just taking the edge off with a tablet or laughing gas isn't enough. A little something more can help, but the patient still has to be able to respond to speech and touch. The dentist may have to place medications through an IV line. Dentists primarily use short-acting IV medications such as midazolam, fentanyl, and propofol. The level of sedation can range from mild to moderate to deep, depending on what's required.

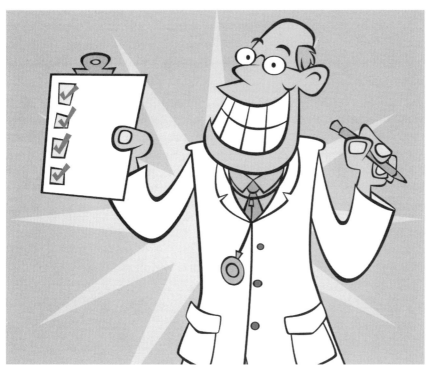

DON'T FORGET TO SEE YOUR DENTIST REGULARLY.

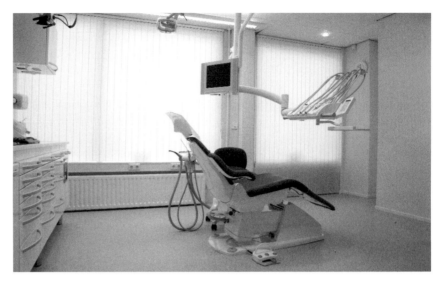

A TYPICAL DENTIST OFFICE

Deep sedation is reserved for complex procedures and to keep patients from moving. A patient under deep sedation is not able to respond appropriately to verbal commands. There is a point where deep sedation borders on general anesthesia. In all circumstances where inhaled gases and IV medications are used, vital signs (heart rate, blood pressure, and oxygen level) have to be continuously monitored, an anesthetic record has to be maintained, and emergency equipment (heart defibrillator) has to be readily available. The facility should have an area where patients can be observed and recover from anesthesia.

Totally Out

When a person is unconscious and unresponsive to physical or verbal command, or can't maintain his breathing independently, he is under general anesthesia. A general anesthetic requires monitoring of vital signs, just as it would in a hospital operating room. All oral surgeons are trained in providing general anesthesia. They are the so-called **surgeon-anesthetists**. This type of specialist is especially needed for complex surgical procedures of the jaws, head, and face. As with other situations when general anesthesia is used, a pre-operative evaluation of the patient's medical history is required.

Options and Choices

Most dental procedures—and most people—do not require much more than a local anesthetic injection. Any additional anesthetic should be taken seriously, just as you would prepare for any major surgery.

The world of dentistry is evolving with increased training about anesthesia, better guidelines, new medications, and improved pain control. So putting off going to the dentist may well be a thing of the past. It's a reason to smile!

Rx Prescriptives: Be a Better Consumer

 If you are "the really nervous type" when it comes to visiting the dentist, ask which anesthetic options besides gum numbing are available. _____

_____

 A friend or relative should accompany you home if you have had oral or intravenous anesthetic medication in the dentist's office. _____

_____

 If intravenous anesthetic or inhaled gas (laughing gas) is planned for your care, make sure your dentist is specially trained to administer it. _____

_____

 Review all your health problems before you get general anesthesia for a dental procedure. You should get a full medical exam if you have problems with your heart or lungs or have diabetes. _____

_____

CHAPTERTHIRTEEN {

the "ick" factor:
post-operative nausea and vomiting

Vomiting? It feels, smells, and looks awful—ick! One of the most common concerns people have *before* surgery is whether they will feel nauseous and begin to vomit *after* they wake up from general anesthesia.

Post-operative nausea and vomiting (PONV) is a valid concern, because it can make the entire anesthetic experience seem unpleasant. There may be nothing in your stomach because you faithfully followed the fasting guidelines, but retching is very uncomfortable. And this

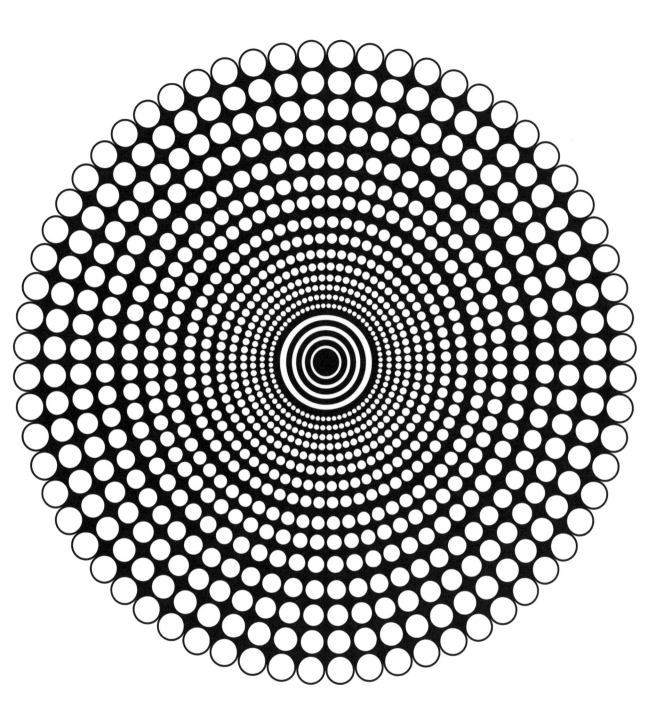

DOES THIS MAKE YOU DIZZY?

may not be only a recovery room problem, because PONV can appear at any time after the operation is complete, and it can even last well beyond the day of surgery.

PONV may have severe consequences for a patient. In some cases, it can lead to increased bleeding (under the skin after a facelift), opening of sutures (after abdominal surgery), and increased pressure inside the eye (of concern after retinal detachment surgery). Prolonged nausea and vomiting can delay discharge from the recovery room, and it is a leading cause of unanticipated hospital admission after surgery.

The Biological Explanation

Various biological mechanisms trigger PONV. The smells, sights, sounds, surrounding motions, and medications—as well as a person's own tendency—all contribute to a feeling of nausea and the urge to vomit.

Nerve signals from the stomach travel to the brain, triggering nausea, retching, and vomiting. For example, **stretch receptors** are activated if the stomach is too full, and **chemical receptors** are activated if something disagreeable is eaten. The so-called **vomiting center** in the brain

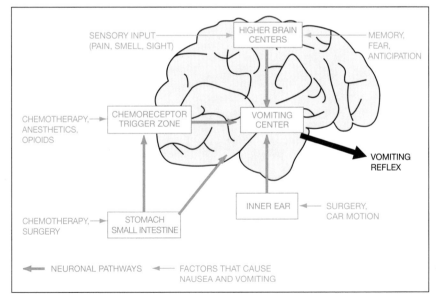

THE VOMITING PATHWAY

is the final common pathway. It receives signals from the gastrointestinal tract, inner ear, and **chemoreceptor** (or chemical receptor) **trigger zone** (CTZ). The CTZ is a special area in the brain that can be stimulated by chemicals in the bloodstream. The vomiting center is also stimulated by complex signals in response to fears, odors, and sights.

When it is activated, the vomiting center induces the act of vomiting. Vomiting involves coordinated action of the salivary glands, respiratory center, gastrointestinal system, and abdominal muscles.

Many different chemical receptors in the brain send nerve signals to the vomiting center. Blocking these receptor sites with **anti-nausea medications** is part of the modern **multimodal** approach to preventing nausea and vomiting. Multimodal means that two or more drugs are used for targeted treatment.

The major factors influencing nausea and vomiting are shown in the vomiting pathway diagram.

Are You Vulnerable?

Anesthesia providers have become good at identifying the types of people who are prone to nausea and vomiting. The people who are at highest risk for PONV:

- Females
- Non-smokers
- Those with a history of motion sickness (car sickness) or prior PONV
- Those who need opioids (morphine, fentanyl) for post-operative pain control

The incidence of PONV increases in children after the age of three if surgery is longer than thirty minutes, after eye surgery, or if a relative is prone to PONV.

The higher the number of these risk factors for PONV, the higher the chance of PONV. The incidences of PONV with the presence of zero, one, two, three, or all four of the risk factors are approximately 10 percent, 20 percent, 40 percent, 60 percent, and 80 percent, respectively.

Other factors associated with an increased risk of PONV are inhaled anesthetic gases, nitrous oxide (laughing gas), dehydration, and long general anesthetic procedures.

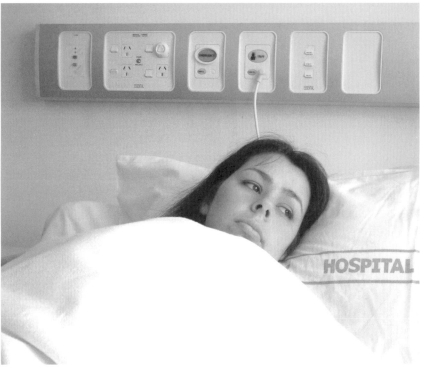

TAKE IT EASY.

The Type of Anesthesia Matters!

Besides the factors described above, certain types of anesthesia may contribute to PONV. For example, if a general anesthetic is not absolutely required, a regional anesthetic or monitored anesthesia care (MAC) can be used. PONV is less common with MAC and regional anesthesia.

But when general anesthesia is used, the anesthesiologist can make modifications for moderate- to high-risk patients. A milk-like injectable anesthetic called **propofol**, used for putting patients to sleep, also helps prevent vomiting. The use of propofol as a part of **total intravenous anesthesia** (TIVA, or no-gas anesthesia) helps reduce PONV.

During general anesthesia, avoiding the use of nitrous oxide, providing adequate hydration, using propofol, and minimizing opioid use can also lower the chances of PONV in people who are at risk.

After some operations, pain may be controlled with medications such as non-steroidal anti-inflammatory drugs (NSAIDs) instead of opioids (narcotics such as morphine). (See chapter 7 for more information on pain management.) Supplementing oxygen after a procedure can also improve the patient's sense of well-being.

The Medications Matter, Too

Anesthesiologists today take a multimodal approach to minimize the likelihood of PONV. Modern-day **prophylaxis** (preventive) drugs for PONV are very effective. They have become a routine part of anesthetic practice. But these medications are not recommended for everyone. Patients who benefit most from **anti-emetics** (drugs used to treat or prevent nausea and vomiting) are those who have a number of risk factors for PONV.

 You may ask to receive these medications if you are prone to nausea and vomiting. The anesthesiologist will be happy to talk this over with you.

PanchLines

Dr. Dhar Notes: Helping the Most Vulnerable Patients

New drugs to combat PONV are always being developed. The latest PONV agent, aprepitant, is a type of receptor blocker. It is taken as a tablet before surgery. Clinical trials have shown the drug to be very effective against nausea and vomiting. This medication is valuable for high-risk patients and for cases in which PONV would be especially ugly and distressing, such as when the jaw is wired shut after dental or facial surgery.

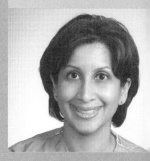

The anti-emetic drugs block receptors (target sites) in the brain, so signals are not sent to the vomiting center. The main prophylaxis drugs are serotonin receptor blockers and dexamethasone. Odansetron (Zofran) is a popular serotonin receptor blocker. It can be taken as a tablet before surgery or given intravenously during a procedure. There are many serotonin receptor blockers available on the market in the United States, such as granisetron and dolasetron. A long-acting serotonin blocker, polanosetron, is undergoing trials as a PONV prevention agent. Dexamethasone is a steroid that is often given with serotonin receptor blockers. Combination anti-emetic prophylaxis drug treatments can reduce the incidence of PONV. For example, using a serotonin receptor blocker *and* dexamethasone is better than using one agent only.

Even with prophylaxis, some patients still experience symptoms of nausea and vomiting. Let's say a person is nauseated despite receiving a serotonin receptor blocker. This is when rescue treatment is necessary. In this situation, "rescue" means using alternative drugs if the initial drug was not 100 percent effective. That is, the current medical guidelines recommend using a drug aimed at a different receptor in the brain. Repeating doses of dexamethasone is not recommended. Large-scale research studies are focusing on different drug combinations and long-acting anti-emetic agents that can work well after surgery is over.

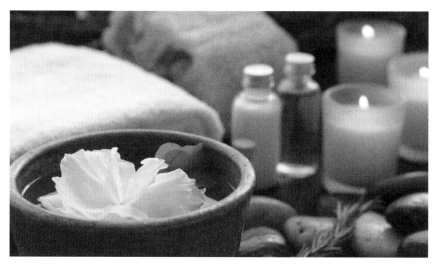

ALTERNATIVE THERAPIES MAY WORK, TOO.

That Queasy Feeling

All of us have experienced nausea at some point. That feeling may have nothing to do with anesthesia. Nausea is a normal physical reaction to something that provokes a queasy sensation in your stomach. Different things trigger the urge to vomit in different people: seasickness, food poisoning, morning sickness, stomach flu, vertigo, or antiretroviral (HIV) medications.

It is important to stay nourished and hydrated even if you are experiencing nausea and vomiting. The best thing to do is eat small, frequent meals, avoiding dairy products, greasy foods, spices, and high-fat meals. As you start to feel better, you can progress to fiber-rich foods such as banana, rice, applesauce, and toast.

Your doctor may advise you to continue taking your medications despite nausea. You may wonder whether you should take your medicines again if you vomit after taking the dose. If you haven't noticed the pills coming back up, the medications are still in your system.

Help Yourself

Patients often try to "self-manage" post-operative nausea and vomiting despite their doctor's orders—they don't take their pain medication, they avoid physical activity, or they take food and liquids before the recommended time. Not taking your pain medication may leave you nausea-free, but it can also extend your recovery time. In addition, severe pain itself may lead to nausea. Limiting your physical activity can also slow the healing process. And eating a meal too early after general anesthesia can lead to vomiting.

Fortunately, there are some things you can do to decrease nausea and vomiting:

- Inhaling the aroma of essential oils such as peppermint and spearmint suppresses nausea.
- Acupressure and acupuncture involve gentle pressure or placement of thin needles on various points along the skin, according to the body's "energy channels" (**meridians**).

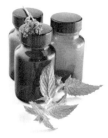

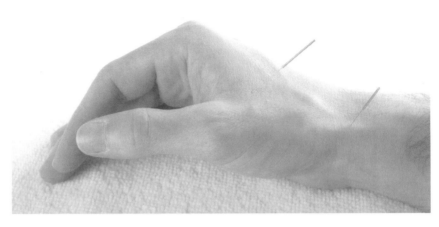

ACUPUNCTURE MAY HELP RELIEVE NAUSEA.

Mild nausea may be relieved by using your middle and index fingers to press firmly down on the groove between the two large tendons on the inside of your wrist that start at the base of your palm. Stimulation of these sites releases chemicals in the brain that inhibit the vomiting center. Acupuncture also decreases acid secretion in the stomach.

- Music therapy has been shown to have a positive effect in recovery. Turn it on!
- The use of relaxation techniques such as yoga and deep breathing exercises can reduce anxiety and curb post-operative nausea.

Comforting Teamwork

Remember, the job to control nausea and vomiting starts before surgery and continues well afterward. You now know in what ways your anesthesiologist is working to avoid the distress of PONV—and how you personally can contribute to your care and comfortable recovery!

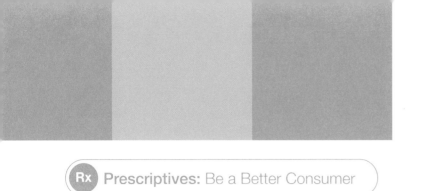

Rx Prescriptives: Be a Better Consumer

☐ Let your anesthesiologist know if you are prone to motion sickness. _____

_____

☐ Ask your anesthesiologist to use anti-nausea medication if you are concerned about feeling sick after surgery. _____

_____

☐ Take a whiff of a fragrance with an anti-nausea property. Fresh lavender, mint, or orange can calm that queasy feeling. _____

_____

☐ Try a ginger-based product to combat nausea, such as ginger snaps, ginger ale, or capsules. _____

_____

☐ Try an anti-nausea wristband. These bands are worn on both wrists and exert a constant gentle pressure over the inner wrist on the acupressure point called nei-kuan. _____

_____

CHAPTERFOURTEEN

awake? aware?
taking care

The idea of remaining awake and aware during surgery *despite being under general anesthesia* is some people's deepest fear. The extremely unusual cases of someone being awake and feeling pain during surgery—while appearing to be totally unconscious and having no way to alert the doctors—have received a huge amount of media attention. Medical TV shows, Web sites, documentaries, and mainstream movies have frequently highlighted the subject.

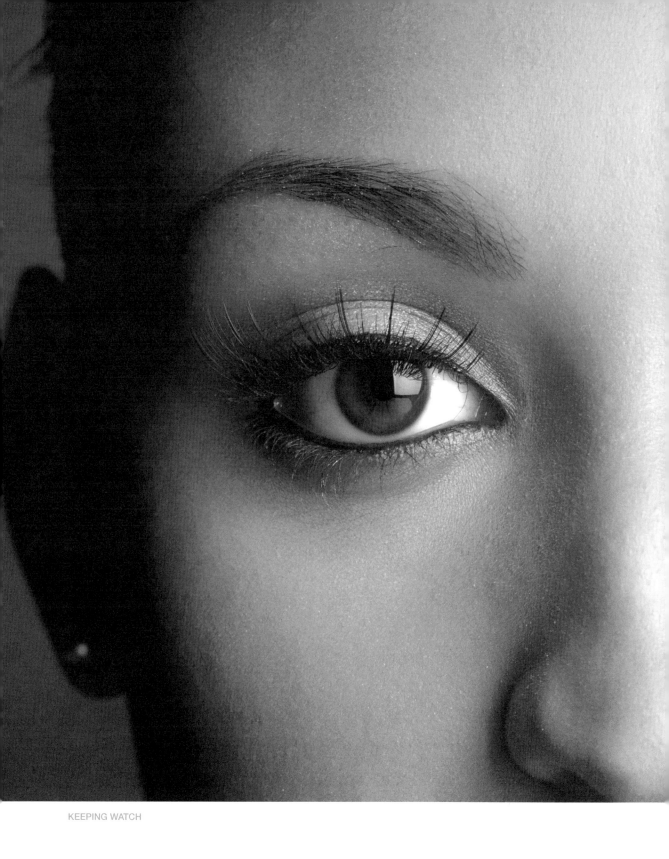

You may even have purchased this book because of concern that this could happen to you or a loved one.

But you can rest easy. The phenomenon is very uncommon.

Distinctions in the Mind

A task force under the American Society of Anesthesiologists (ASA) gathered information from major research studies, expert consultants, case reports, open forums, and surveys. The purpose of the task force was to identify risk factors for "awareness during surgery" and to promote preventive strategies and practices.

The ASA task force report clarified a number of definitions to better help understand the phenomenon of awareness. **Consciousness** means a person is able to process information from his surroundings. **Recall** is the ability to retrieve stored information from memory and report things or events that took place in the past. **Intra-operative awareness** means a patient remains or becomes conscious while under general anesthesia; he may or may not have the ability to recall specific events.

Interestingly, awareness is not always associated with recall. A good analogy of awareness without recall is an instance when a person is drunk. He may be aware of his surroundings at the time, but later he has no specific recall of what he said or did. While drunk, his brain simply did not register any memory of the events.

The Awareness Spectrum

There is a wide range, or spectrum, of awareness circumstances. At one end of the spectrum are surgical situations where patients consent to remain conscious. For example, an "awake" craniotomy requires the patient to speak coherently while the surgeon identifies areas in the brain involved in language or speech. The patient is awake but not in pain, as the brain itself does not have pain nerve fibers.

Examples in the middle of the spectrum are procedures that are performed under monitored anesthesia care (MAC) or under regional anesthesia. (See chapter 2 for more information on the types of anesthesia.) A breast nodule can be removed under local anesthesia with sedation (MAC). During MAC anesthesia, the depth of sedation is based on surgical

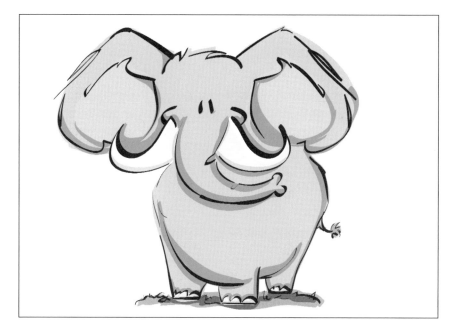

AN ELEPHANT NEVER FORGETS.

and patient requirements. Regional anesthesia may be used to remove a thyroid gland; only the nerves of the neck are anesthetized, and the patient is sedated. In both of these situations, a brief awakening may occur—if the level of surgical stimulation increases, or if a higher dose of sedative is needed.

The recall of events during this period can be minimized or prevented with drugs that cause amnesia. Amnesia means a partial or total loss of memory of events. Amnestic medications used in anesthesia prevent new memories from being formed. A drug such as midazolam (Versed, a short-acting benzodiazepine that is related to Valium) is often given to block the patient's memory. Awareness under a MAC or regional anesthetic may occur, but it is not disastrous, because the patient knows beforehand that this might happen. The patient undergoing MAC anesthesia can always ask to be more deeply sedated if he feels uncomfortable or anxious.

The danger end of the awareness spectrum is when a patient *appears* to be unconscious and immobile but is actually conscious—hearing and

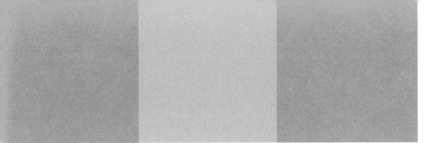

feeling what is happening while under general anesthesia. Patients who have experienced awareness under general anesthesia have reported hearing sounds and conversations, feeling suffocated or paralyzed, and feeling pain. They also have reported feelings of helplessness, powerlessness, anxiety, and panic from the inability to notify the surgical team of what they were experiencing.

What Are the Chances?

Fortunately, intra-operative awareness under general anesthesia is an uncommon occurrence. There is a reported incidence of 0.1 to 0.2 percent among the millions of general anesthetics administered every year. In one study of a large number of patients (over 87,000) at a regional medical center, the incidence of intra-operative awareness under general anesthesia was 0.0068 percent, or 1 per 14,560 patients.

Intra-operative awareness under general anesthesia cannot be readily measured, because recall can only be determined if the patient draws attention to it (that is, reports the incident). Some patients who experience awareness during general anesthesia develop **post-traumatic stress disorder** (PTSD). This can require counseling with a trained therapist.

Another thing to keep in mind is that some reported incidents of recall may actually be remembrance of details upon awakening from general anesthesia or from a semi-awake state in the recovery room.

Dreaming during anesthesia is another issue that requires more research, since it's unclear what its relation is to awareness.

Most anesthesia providers never see a case of intra-operative awareness in their entire career. But as with any anesthetic complication, the key is prevention. However, at this time, there is no single anesthetic technique, monitoring device, or set of circumstances that will absolutely guarantee a lack of awareness and recall under general anesthesia.

Dr. Dhar Explains: What Are You Getting Into?

It is understandable that one of the strongest fears everyone has about "going under" is actually being awake or waking up suddenly in the middle of an operation. A common general anesthetic experience is waking up and asking "When are you starting?" only to hear the answer "It's over, we're done!"

General anesthesia is all about being unconscious and motionless. When the motionless part happens—but the unconsciousness part doesn't happen—that makes a reportable story. Thankfully, this experience is not common. Here are a few facts to remember to help you move forward with surgery.

- During a general anesthetic you expect nothing but total unconsciousness.
- Keep in mind that with some anesthetics such as sedation or blocks you may be able to hear and also speak up. The primary goal here is to be pain-free and relaxed.

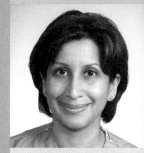

High-Risk Circumstances

Every case of intra-operative awareness during general anesthesia is unintentional. Awareness during anesthesia has been reported after apparently adequate levels of anesthesia have been given. But in the practice of anesthesia, some circumstances may mean some patients are more at risk of experiencing awareness. Studies have identified these high-risk situations. There is more chance of awareness in certain procedures (heart bypass surgery), patient populations (pregnant women for cesarean section), health conditions (critically ill patients), and surgery performed under emergency conditions.

The delivery of low concentrations of anesthetic gas has been implicated in some cases of awareness. For example, during an emergency C-section, the anesthesiologist may provide a low level of anesthetic gas until the baby is delivered—there is a risk of awareness because the mother is given a lower level of gas to avoid anesthetizing the baby.

Light anesthesia may be needed in situations of heavy blood loss, low blood pressure, or poor heart function. The concentration of anesthetic gas may need to be lowered because routine levels may not be tolerated by the patient. A history of awareness during surgery may also put a patient at future risk for intra-operative awareness.

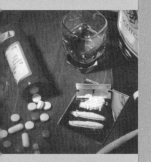

Memory Management

Some people simply need more anesthetic to block memory because each person's dose requirement is different. But it is important to emphasize that chronic use of alcohol, narcotics (such as heroin), amphetamines, and cocaine may increase the dose requirement of anesthetic agents. A complication can occur if the anesthesiologist does not know about the patient's drug or alcohol use. This is yet another reason why patients should be up-front with their anesthesiologist about their lifestyle habits.

Technology for Protection

Equipment or Human Judgment?

Equipment problems leading to intra-operative awareness rarely occur today. Multiple alarms on the anesthesia machine protect against mishaps (like use of an empty canister of anesthetic gas). Newer gas canisters are equipped with level alarms.

Such alarms are very helpful, of course, but a vigilant anesthesiologist is your best protection. She knows to perform repeat equipment checks between cases.

Computers cannot fully replace human interpretation of vital signs and clinical judgment. That's why the anesthesiologist so carefully watches her patient for signs such as movement, perspiration, tearing of the eyes, and increasing heart rate and blood pressure. Sudden movement is an important sign that a patient is under-anesthetized. A good

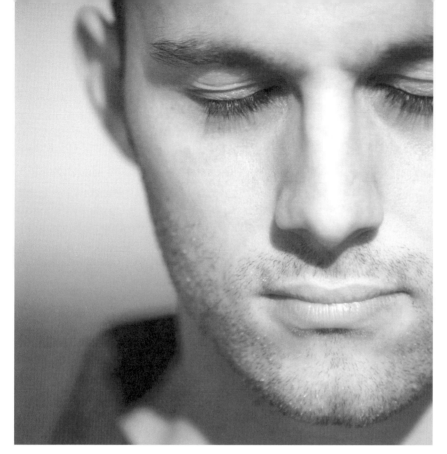

THINK OF YOUR FAVORITE VACATION.

anesthesiologist is *constantly* watching for such telltale signs and adjusting the level of anesthesia as needed.

Besides being a good doctor, what more can an anesthesiologist do to prevent awareness? New technology has been developed to assess **depth of anesthesia** in a patient who is under general anesthesia. The technology uses computer algorithms and is frequently used as part of monitoring practices.

Among the monitors that keep watch on depth of anesthesia, the **bispectral index (BIS) monitor** (from Aspect Medical Systems) has been the most extensively evaluated. With the BIS, a large Band-Aid–like adhesive strip is attached to the patient's forehead. The strip primarily detects electrical activity in the brain and sends the information to the monitor. A computer algorithm inside the monitor interprets the data, and the screen displays a number between 0 and 100. The idea behind this is: the greater the depth of anesthesia, the less the total electrical activity,

hence the lower the number. A fully awake and alert person has a reading of 100. A number in the range of 40 to 60 reflects a low probability of consciousness under general anesthesia.

Should Anesthesia Depth Monitors Always Be Used?

Research studies have compared the incidence of awareness with and without the BIS monitor in patients under general anesthesia. The studies show mixed outcomes. Some studies have shown that using the BIS monitor may help reduce the incidence of awareness in high-risk patients (such as trauma, heart surgery, C-section, chronic drug use, and a history of awareness). But it is important to note that the BIS number is affected by many variables that can erroneously increase or decrease the number. A study in the *New England Journal of Medicine* evaluated a patient population considered to be at high risk for anesthesia awareness, or inadvertent waking during surgery. Researchers compared BIS-guided anesthesia care to an older device that tracks the level of anesthetic gas exhaled by patients and found a similar occurrence of awareness in the two groups. Although controversial, the study did not demonstrate target BIS ranges to eliminate the chance of awareness.

At the time of this writing, *routine* depth of anesthesia monitoring is not considered the "standard of care" by the American Society of Anesthesiologists. The ASA recommends that it be used on a case-by-case

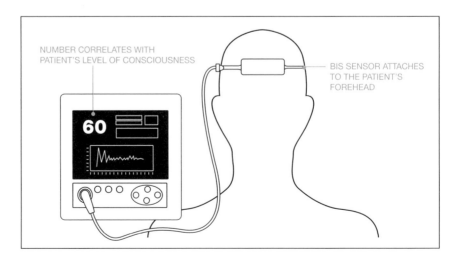

NUMBER CORRELATES WITH
PATIENT'S LEVEL OF CONSCIOUSNESS

BIS SENSOR ATTACHES
TO THE PATIENT'S
FOREHEAD

60

A BIS MONITOR

basis. No monitor has been proven to eliminate awareness or has been established as the standard.

Many anesthesiologists in the United States, however, do regularly use the BIS monitor as a complementary tool to help guide the dose of anesthetic. The decision to use a monitor is based on the choice of the anesthesia provider and on patient risk factors. Prevention of awareness ultimately depends on good clinical judgment on the part of the anesthesiologist, among other things. Every general anesthetic has to be carefully adjusted for a patient's personalized requirements.

The Anesthesia Awareness Registry

Any case of awareness needs to be documented, because the phenomenon is very serious. If this happens to you, you should report your experience to those who have taken care of you. The case should be reported in the national Anesthesia Awareness Registry (www.awaredb.org), which seeks greater understanding about the causes of this problem.

Patients interested in reporting to the registry fill out a short questionnaire and have an opportunity to discuss their experiences in more detail with a member of the study team for the Awareness Registry. Some patients will be asked to submit copies of portions of their medical records to the registry.

The goals of the Anesthesia Awareness Registry are to help the professional community understand

- Why awareness occurs
- How to prevent it in the future
- How to help anesthesiologists and other physicians respond better to patients and help them if awareness does occur

You Really Can Rest Easy!

So where does that leave us? To summarize: intra-operative awareness is a real and frightening phenomenon—but it is an uncommon experience. Sensationalism by the media is entertainment, but far removed from reality. You should not be deterred from having necessary surgery because of the remote possibility of awareness. Anesthesia itself is a miracle that allows everyone to have fulfilling lives. If you are concerned about it, discuss the matter with your anesthesiologist. Ask the doctor how your anesthetic levels will be monitored during surgery.

Top professionals in the world of anesthesia are actively seeking and developing ways to prevent intra-operative awareness from ever occurring. You can have faith in your anesthesiologist to be fully informed about the issue and to do her best to make sure it doesn't happen to you. You can indeed literally "rest easy" while you are under!

Rx Prescriptives: Be a Better Consumer

☐ If you are getting general anesthesia, ask if a depth of anesthesia monitor (e.g., the BIS monitor) will be used. _____

_____

☐ Let your anesthesia provider know of any of the following, which could place you at high risk of awareness:

    ☐ A previous history of awareness _____

    ☐ A history of difficult intubation_____

    ☐ A history of substance use/abuse_____

    ☐ High-dose opioids taken for chronic pain_____

☐ Ask if your anesthesia will be mostly intravenous drugs instead of a gas. If so, you will need the addition of memory blockers (midazolam) in your anesthetic.

_____

☐ Let your anesthesia provider know if you specifically remember anything during a general anesthetic._____

_____

☐ Rest and relax before any procedure. High levels of anxiety may require more anesthetic to keep you under. _____

_____

references
and tools
{

anesthesia through the ages

Try to imagine being operated on without anesthesia! There was a time when anesthesia, as we know it today, had not developed as a branch of medicine. As a result of people's very reasonable fear of pain and death, surgery was avoided unless absolutely essential, such as to remove a badly mangled leg. If someone *did* have to have surgery, the patient might first drink large amounts of alcohol, as it was a lot easier for the surgeon to operate on an inebriated patient. Several people would have to hold the person down with all their strength so the operation could proceed.

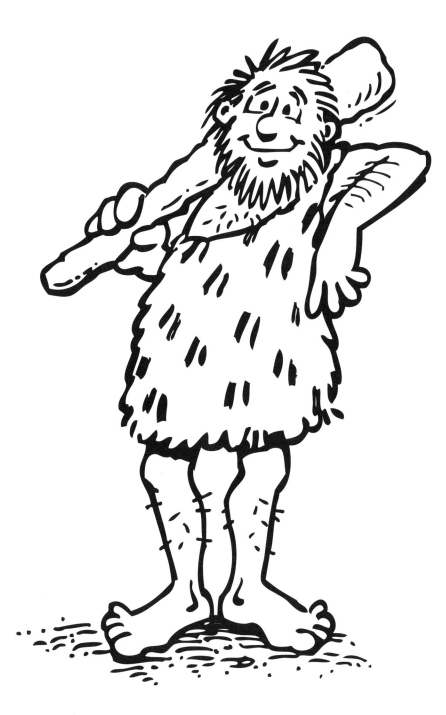

STONE AGE ANESTHESIA

The surgeon then had to work quickly to shorten the period of agony. Surgery was primitive, painful, dirty, and risky. If patients survived the operation, they often later died of infection.

Attitudes about pain were different in the past. Before modern anesthesia, pain was thought of as an inevitable part of surgery, and it had to be met with courage. Most people did not even imagine that pain could be prevented. Today, even the pinprick of a needle insertion into your gums can be avoided with a topical numbing cream.

Old School

Some form of anesthesia was practiced by all ancient civilizations. Most of the concoctions were inhaled as vapors or consumed. The purpose was to induce sleep, dull the mind, and hopefully calm the frightened patient. Combinations of wine, opium, marijuana, mandrake, and jimsonweed are mentioned throughout ancient texts of many cultures. The opium poppy may have been used by prehistoric peoples; it found its way into Egypt by the second century A.D. Peruvian Indians knew of the coca shrub—the source of cocaine, which is a local anesthetic. Other techniques that were practiced in the past include hypnotism and bleeding patients to the point of unconsciousness.

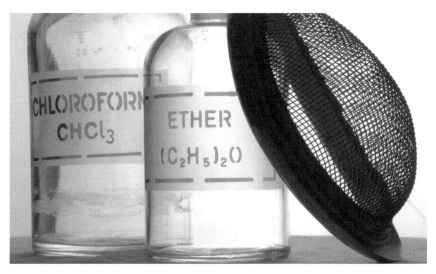

YESTERDAY'S COMMON GASES

None of these techniques were very reliable. Alcohol and opium were practical, but many people died from overdose. It seems these "solutions" simply put patients in a foggy state of mind where the dread of surgery was more tolerable.

Modern medicine's anesthetic tools and sophisticated surgical techniques took centuries to develop. Surgery, once done in extreme haste to minimize pain and patient movement, can now be done with time and care.

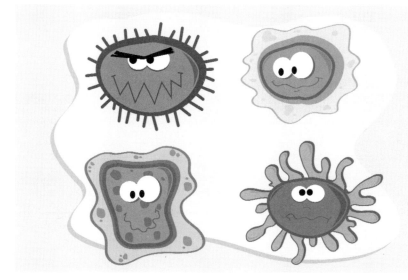

GERMS AROUND US

Steps in the Right Direction

In the 1800s, Louis Pasteur discovered that bacteria caused disease and infection. This discovery has saved vast numbers of people who have had surgery since then.

The idea of making every surface in the operating area safe from infection—**antiseptic**—was established by Joseph Lister in 1867. He sprayed the operating rooms and cleaned surgical wounds with carbolic acid (phenol). This made an incredible difference in the infection rate. Today all instruments, gowns, and gloves are sterile—**aseptic**. Hair is covered and masks are worn to further decrease the chance of an infection passing from the surgical team to the patient.

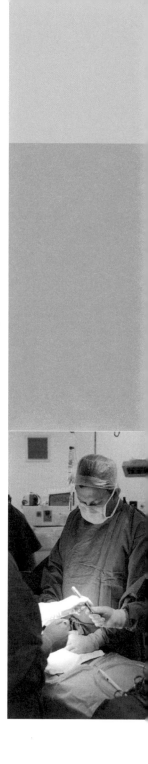

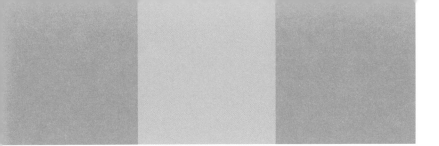

Our average lifespan has expanded in the past century because of preventive medicine, early detection of disease—and the appropriate use of anesthesia. It is because of anesthesia that surgeons can so deftly perform their craft.

Anesthesia Time Line

Here are some highlights of how modern anesthesia evolved through the contributions of physicians, dentists, and scientists.

1772 British clergyman and chemist Joseph Priestley discovers nitrous oxide (laughing gas).

1800 Humphry Davy, a British chemist and physicist, experiments with nitrous oxide on himself. He notes that inhaling the gas causes intoxication, euphoria, and decreased pain, and suggests it could be used during surgery.

1831 Samuel Guthrie, a U.S. physician, creates a new alcohol-like substance later known as chloroform. Independently, two other chemists—Eugène Soubeiran in France and Justus von Liebig in Germany—also announce the discovery of chloroform. It is used as an anesthetic a few years later.

1842 Crawford W. Long, a physician, uses ether to anesthetize a patient.

1844 Horace Wells, a dentist, has one of his own teeth extracted under nitrous oxide.

1846 William Morton, a dentist and pupil of Horace Wells, arranges the first public demonstration of surgery using ether.

1847 James Simpson, an obstetrician in Scotland, reduces pain during childbirth with chloroform, bringing it into practical use.

1853 British physician John Snow administers inhaled chloroform to Queen Victoria during childbirth. A humanitarian attitude toward labor pain begins to set in all over the world.

1874 Pierre-Cyprien Ore introduces the practice of injecting medication directly into the blood for general anesthesia instead of breathing a gas.

1876 Joseph Thomas Clover develops a dispenser to deliver anesthetic gases like chloroform and ether.

1884 Carl Koller demonstrates that cocaine can be used as a local anesthetic. William Halsted and Karl Schleich promote the concept of placing cocaine around nerves and under the skin to block pain.

1898 August Bier refines spinal anesthesia. Its use is widespread by the 1920s.

1900 Harvey Cushing promotes safety in anesthesia by monitoring a patient's blood pressure during an operation and by keeping an anesthetic record.

1902 Franz Kunz introduces oxygen and anesthetic gases through a tube placed in the windpipe (trachea).

1934 John Lundy is credited with developing the first post-anesthesia care unit (PACU) in the world at St. Mary's Hospital in Rochester, Minnesota.

1942 Harold Griffith and G. Enid Johnson introduce curare, a hunting poison used by South American Indians, as a muscle relaxant to make surgery easier.

1950–today Great strides are made, including the development of anesthesia machines and computerized monitoring equipment; fast-onset, short-acting anesthetics with fewer side effects; and patient-controlled analgesia pumps. Research is being done to understand how anesthesia differs from sleep and to locate sites in the brain where these drugs work.

everyday medications used for anesthesia

These are the most common medications used every day to deliver anesthesia. They are combined in light doses to create "cocktails" for sedation or combined in heavier doses for general anesthesia. Except for the gases, all of the medications are in liquid form and are given through an intravenous line. Certain opioids (narcotics) can be used for spinal and epidural anesthesia.

Medication	Generic name	Profile
Benzodiazepine		Sedative. Reduces anxiety. Blocks memory formation.
Versed	midazolam	Just like Valium, but short acting.
Opioid (narcotic)		Pain killer.
	morphine	The standard for comparing the strength of other opioids.
Sublimaze	fentanyl	Most common opioid used in anesthesia.
Sufenta	sufentanil	Extremely potent opioid.
Alfenta	alfentanil	Short-acting opioid.
Ultiva	remifentanil	Ultra-short-acting opioid.
Induction agent		A knockout drug. When given as a large one-time dose, it starts a general anesthetic.
Diprivan	propofol	A sedative when given in small doses. Could be painful during injection. Looks like milk.

Medication	Generic name	Profile
Pentothal	thiopental	A fast-onset and short-acting barbiturate.
Amidate	etomidate	Used for frail patients (very old or with low blood pressure).
	ketamine	Related to PCP, thus it can have psychotropic side effects in small doses (referred to as "Special K" on the street).
Anesthetic gas		Inhaled through a mask, a breathing tube (endotracheal tube), or an LMA. Maintains unconsciousness, prevents movement, blocks memory formation and pain.
Ultane	sevoflurane	
Suprane	desflurane	
	nitrous oxide	Commonly known as "laughing gas."
Muscle relaxant		Used during general anesthesia to prevent movement so the surgeon can operate.
	succinylcholine	
Nimbex	cisatracurium	
Zemuron	rocuronium	

glossary

accreditation A third-party verification that a facility meets requirements for patient safety, proper functioning of equipment, and credentialing of persons working there.

airway management A term broadly including all the maneuvers and devices used to maintain and ensure unobstructed oxygenation and removal of exhaled carbon dioxide in a patient. It includes placement of devices such as an endotracheal tube or laryngeal mask airway.

airway management device Any device used to ensure breathing and oxygenation (optimize level of oxygen in the blood), such as a face mask. A variety of devices aid in placement of a breathing tube (endotracheal tube) in the windpipe (trachea); for example, a laryngoscope, fiberoptic scope, GlideScope, and Airtraq.

ambulatory surgery A procedure that allows a patient to go home the same day after an operation or procedure.

amnesia Loss of memory.

analgesia Pain control; absence of pain.

anesthesia assistant (AA) A non-physician health professional who works under the direction of licensed anesthesiologists to implement anesthesia care plans.

anesthesia machine A machine used to support the administration of anesthesia. It is integrated with an oxygen and anesthetic gas delivery system and a ventilator (breathing machine) to support patient breathing.

anesthesia resident A licensed physician receiving training in anesthesiology in a hospital. The training period ranges from three to four years after medical school.

anesthesiologist A licensed physician who practices anesthesiology in a hospital or surgical facility. This person may be a medical physician, dentist, or oral/maxillofacial surgeon.

anesthetic plan A mental plan or discussion about the type of anesthetic and care a patient is to receive during surgery.

anesthetic record A detailed record of the events during surgery. It includes information about the anesthetic, surgical procedure, vital signs, fluids administered, and any pertinent events.

anti-emetic (anti-nausea medication) A drug used to prevent or treat nausea and vomiting.

antiseptic Something that discourages the growth of microorganisms like bacteria.

arterial line A catheter placed directly into an artery that allows continuous measurement of blood pressure and permits blood sampling.

aseptic Free from contaminating germs or bacteria. Sterile.

aspiration The entry of stomach contents, secretions, or foreign material into the trachea or lungs. This can cause serious breathing problems, lower blood oxygen levels, infection, and lung damage.

attending physician anesthesiologist See anesthesiologist.

bacteria Microscopic life forms, many of which cause infection and disease. They can be killed with antibiotics.

bispectral index (BIS) monitor A "depth of anesthesia" monitor that continually analyzes a patient's brain waves to assess the level of consciousness. The monitor displays a dimensionless number from 0 to 100. The greater the depth of general anesthesia, the lower the number. A number between 40 and 60 is believed to coincide with a low probability of awareness during general anesthesia.

block failure A situation when patchy areas of the body continue to have sensation or movement after a spinal, epidural, or peripheral nerve block anesthetic. This happens because of uneven distribution of anesthetic.

blood pressure cuff An automated device that measures a patient's blood pressure.

board-certified A term applied to a physician or nurse who has passed a nationally standardized exam in a medical specialty or area of practice.

body mass index (BMI) A number calculated from a person's weight and height as a gauge of total body fat.

bolus A fixed dose or one-time dose of medication.

capnograph A machine that measures the amount of carbon dioxide in each exhaled breath.

catheter A hollow, flexible tube that can be inserted into a blood vessel or body cavity.

central line A catheter placed in a large vein, most commonly in the neck up to the large veins entering the heart. It can be used to measure the amount of fluid in the body (the central venous pressure) and provide a route to give medications, blood, and other fluids.

central venous pressure A reflection of the amount of fluid in the body. A low value can result from dehydration or blood loss. A high value can result from poor pumping action of the heart, with blood backing up in the circulation (heart failure).

cerebrospinal fluid (CSF) A clear fluid produced in the brain that circulates around the surface and in the cavities of the brain and spinal cord. It acts as a cushion and shock absorber, provides a path for excretion of harmful substances, and serves as a vehicle for chemical messengers to circulate in the nervous system.

certified registered nurse anesthetist (CRNA) An advanced-practice nurse with a master's degree who is specially trained in anesthesiology. CRNAs are capable of providing anesthesia for every type of surgery or procedure.

cesarean section (C-section) A surgical procedure in which a baby is delivered through the abdominal wall and uterus.

chart A file containing all the information regarding a patient such as medical history, current medical issues, laboratory data, test results, list of medications, and treatment plan.

chemical receptors A target site in the body where chemicals in the blood (drugs, anesthetics, neurotransmitters) can attach and then either stimulate or inhibit functions in an organ.

chemoreceptor trigger zone (CTZ) An area of the brain that receives input from chemicals in the blood (anesthetic drugs, opioids) and then sends signals to the vomiting center to initiate nausea and vomiting.

circulating nurse A nurse in the operating room who is responsible for patient safety and who provides any assistance to the scrub nurse, anesthesia provider, or surgeon.

consciousness A state in which a person is responsive and aware of his surroundings.

continuous peripheral nerve block A regional anesthesia technique in which a catheter is placed near nerves supplying a part of the body. The catheter is connected to a pump delivering pain medication (local anesthetic and/or narcotic).

cosmetic surgery Plastic surgery for an aesthetic purpose and done as an elective procedure.

defibrillator An electrical device used to restore a regular heart rhythm. Commonly called "shock paddles."

dehydration A condition in which the body has lost an excessive amount of water. Doctors refer to dehydrated patients as "being dry."

deliberate hypothermia Intentionally lowering the temperature of the body to protect the brain and heart during surgery.

dental/oral surgeon A dentist who has an additional four years of training in surgery of the head, jaw, and neck. Also called an oral/maxillofacial surgeon.

depth of anesthesia The level of depression of the brain and spinal cord activity produced by anesthetics. A measure of loss of consciousness and awareness.

diagnostic procedure A test or an exam done to identify the cause of symptoms or of a condition or to distinguish one disease from another. It can be a blood test for cholesterol levels or a mammogram to evaluate a breast lump.

dural puncture A hole inadvertently made in one of the membranes surrounding the spinal cord. It leads to a cerebrospinal fluid leak and may result in a spinal headache.

elective surgery A procedure that a patient chooses to have, not one that is considered urgent or required.

electrocardiogram (EKG) A graphic recording of the electrical activity of the heart produced by an electrocardiograph. It provides information regarding the rate, rhythm, and electrical conduction of the heart.

electroencephalograph (EEG) A device that produces a graphic recording (electroencephalogram) of the electrical activity of the brain. Recorded brain wave patterns are used to assess changes in blood flow during surgery on blood vessels supplying the brain.

emergence The end of general anesthesia, when the anesthetic is stopped or reversed and the patient awakens.

endotracheal tube (ETT) A hollow tube made of plastic with an inflatable cuff at the end. It is placed in the trachea (windpipe) through the mouth or nose to allow delivery of oxygen and anesthetic gases. Also called a breathing tube. It is connected to the anesthesia circuit, which leads to the anesthesia machine. It allows delivery of oxygen and anesthetic gases into the lungs.

epidural anesthetic A form of regional anesthesia where a catheter is inserted into the epidural space surrounding the spinal cord. Local anesthetics and/or opioids are injected to numb the body from the waist down (abdomen and legs).

epidural blood patch A small amount of blood taken under sterile conditions from an arm vein is injected through an epidural needle above the site of a dural puncture. This blood clots and seals the hole in the dura, preventing further leak of cerebrospinal fluid. It is used for the treatment of spinal headache.

evoked potential An electrical response detected in the brain or spinal cord elicited by stimulation of a nerve in the leg or arm. Potentials can also be detected in a nerve after stimulating a location in the brain.

face mask A clear plastic device that sits snugly over a patient's mouth and nose. The top end is connected to the anesthesia circuit, which leads to the anesthesia machine. It allows delivery of oxygen and anesthetic gases into the lungs.

fiberoptic bronchoscope (camera) A flexible, long, thin camera containing optical fibers that transmit light at one end, with an eyepiece to look through the device at the other end. The scope can be placed through the mouth or nose and advanced into the trachea. It can be used to place endotracheal tubes.

gastroesophageal reflux disease (GERD) A condition where there is abnormal backflow of stomach juices and acid up into the tube that leads from the throat to the stomach (esophagus). One of the symptoms is heartburn at least twice a week.

general anesthesia A type of anesthesia that consists of loss of consciousness, amnesia (loss of memory), lack of pain, and/or immobility (inability

to move). Also referred to as "completely going to sleep" or "being completely out."

hypnosis Loss of consciousness.

hypnotics Medications that are calmative and induce sleep, such as propofol.

induction The beginning of general anesthesia when the patient goes from a conscious state to an unconscious state.

intensive care Continuous and closely monitored health care for critically ill patients. Examples of such patients are people who have had a heart attack, patients after extensive surgery, or victims of severe car accidents.

intra-operative awareness A state when a patient has not had enough general anesthetic and can feel or hear what is happening during surgery. The person may not be able to move in response.

intravenous (IV) Into a vein.

intubation The act of placing a breathing tube (endotracheal tube) into the windpipe (trachea).

labor suite (labor ward) The area in the hospital where pregnant woman give birth.

local anesthesia Chemicals that reversibly block transmission of impulses in nerves. Sensations in the area supplied by the nerves are numbed. The strength and dosage of the anesthetic can be changed to block movement in the lower body or limbs. These types of anesthetics are used in all forms of regional anesthesia: local, spinal, epidural, and peripheral nerve blocks. Although there are many types of local anesthetic, a common name is "novocaine."

lockout interval Used in patient-controlled analgesia machines to prevent a patient from repeating a dose of medication for a set period of time.

maintenance In all forms of anesthesia (general, regional, sedation), continuation of the anesthetic.

malignant hyperthermia (MH) An uncommon genetic condition in which certain anesthetics (inhaled gas or succinylcholine) can cause extremely high body temperature and muscle rigidity. It is fatal if not treated promptly.

mechanical ventilation The use of a machine to take over active breathing for a patient. The machine is called a ventilator. *See also* Ventilation.

medical clearance A document provided by a patient's primary care physician or a specialist documenting pertinent health information and test results. The information is used to guide the anesthesiologist about special requirements or health issues the patient may have during surgery.

medi-spa A spa location that offers treatments such as laser and pulsed light procedures, micro-dermabrasion, chemical facial peels, photofacial, Botox, and chemical fillers (Restylane, Cosmoderm). The location is supervised by a licensed health-care professional.

meninges Thin layers of membrane (tissue) that envelop the brain and spinal cord. They consist of three layers: the dura mater, the arachnoid mater, and the pia mater. The primary function of the meninges and of the cerebrospinal fluid is to protect the brain and spinal cord.

meridians The basis for acupuncture/acupressure. These are pathways throughout the surface of the body where energy, called qi, travels. The flow of qi is responsible for maintaining good health. Blockage, deficiencies, or disturbances in qi cause health problems. Localized stimulation of specific points (needle, pressure) re-establishes the flow of qi.

monitored anesthesia care (MAC) Sometimes this term is used interchangeably with "twilight sleep" or "conscious sedation." Sedation is created by carefully titrating combinations of medications. Deep levels of sedation border on a state of general anesthesia. Although amnesia (loss of memory) is common during this type of anesthesia, it is not the primary goal of the anesthesia provider.

monitors An electronic device incorporating a computer that interprets, displays, and records a function inside the body.

multimodal An approach using two or more drugs to achieve a goal.

muscle relaxation A condition rendered by particular anesthetic drugs called muscle relaxants. After receiving the medication the patient cannot move, so it must be accompanied by unconsciousness.

narcotic Any medication that relieves pain. Side effects include slowed breathing, sleepiness, and euphoria. Also called opioid.

neonates Newborns.

nil per os (NPO) A Latin term used in medicine to mean nothing by mouth. That means no food, liquids, or alcohol can be taken before surgery. Sips of water can be taken with required medications.

nociceptors Nerve endings that send signals up to the brain about feelings of pain from such things as a hot iron, a sharp knife edge, a burn, or a heavy object dropping on your foot.

obstetric anesthesia The branch of anesthesia concerned with relieving the pain of pregnant women in labor for childbirth, natural or surgical (cesarean section).

office-based procedures A non-hospital location, usually a doctor's office.

off-site locations A location outside of the operating room. Examples are a radiology suite or gastroenterology suite.

on-call An assignment where physicians and nurses are required to stay in the hospital or be immediately available for after-hours patient care such as nights, weekends, holidays.

operating room (OR) The location where surgery is done.

opioid Also called narcotics. A drug used to treat pain. Examples are morphine, codeine, fentanyl, and meperidine. Opium is derived from the poppy plant.

outpatient pain clinic A private office run by anesthesiologists specifically geared toward the diagnosis and treatment of pain.

oxygenated Treated, combined, or enriched with oxygen.

patient-controlled analgesia/patient-controlled epidural analgesia (PCA/PCEA) A method of pain control where a programmed automatic pump connected to an intravenous line or epidural catheter delivers pain medication. The patient can press a button if more medication is desired.

pediatric anesthesia The branch of anesthesia concerned with the care of babies and children (up to eighteen years of age).

pediatric anesthesiologist A doctor who specializes in the anesthesia care for children.

perioperative Care rendered to patients before, during, and after surgery.

peripheral nerve block A regional anesthesia technique in which local anesthetics are applied near nerves to block sensation and movement.

physician anesthesiologist See anesthesiologist.

plastic surgery Surgery to remodel, repair, and restore a part of the body for an improved appearance or function.

post-anesthesia care unit (PACU) Recovery room.

post-operative nausea and vomiting (PONV) A common problem after receiving anesthesia. Certain patients are at greater risk than others.

post-traumatic stress disorder (PTSD) An anxiety disorder that develops after a traumatic event. It is characterized by re-experiencing the trauma with nightmares, obsessive thoughts, and flashbacks.

premie Premature infant. An infant born less than thirty-seven weeks after conception.

prophylaxis Preventive treatment or measures.

propofol A short-acting intravenous anesthetic agent that looks like milk. Depending on the dose, it can be used to maintain sedation or induce general anesthesia. It may cause a stinging and burning sensation at the site of injection.

pulmonary artery catheter (PAC) A catheter placed into a large vein in the neck and that enters the heart. It is a diagnostic tool that provides information on the amount of blood in the heart chambers, pumping action of the heart, and effects of heart and blood pressure medications.

pulse oximeter A device that measures the oxygen level in the blood by using a sensor transmitting a red light. The pulse oximeter is commonly attached to a finger. It displays a computerized readout on a monitor screen. The pitch of the beeping sound correlates with the number reading.

recall When a patient has distinct memory of events (sounds, voices, touch) after it was assumed the patient was under general anesthesia and unconscious.

reconstructive plastic surgery A subcategory of plastic surgery geared toward restoration of form and function.

regional anesthesia Anesthesia that affects only a part of the body. It includes spinal, epidural, and nerve blocks. Local anesthetics are used to block nerves controlling sensation and movement.

same-day surgery center A non-hospital or hospital-based facility where a person can go from home to have a surgery or procedure done. If in a hospital, the patient may be required to stay after the surgery.

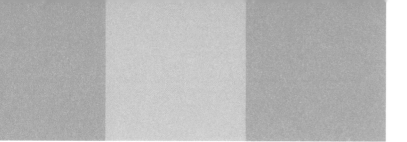

scalpel A surgical knife.

scrub nurse A designated nurse in the operating room who hands over the necessary surgical instruments to the surgeon and helps maintain patient safety. In some procedures he/she may also assist in the surgery. The scrub nurse wears sterile gloves and gown plus a hat and mask.

scrubs Protective cloth or heavy paper garments worn by personnel in the operating room or procedure area. Common colors are green or blue. They are washed in the hospital laundry to prevent outside contamination. Also called scrub suit.

sedation Reduction of anxiety, stress, and fear brought about by anesthetic medications. It may result in sleep with certain doses of anesthetic medication.

sepsis An acute health condition in which there is widespread bacterial infection of the bloodstream and organs.

sleep apnea A problem during sleep characterized by pauses in breathing of at least ten seconds. It is commonly associated with snoring and weight gain.

spinal anesthetic A type of regional anesthesia where local anesthetic is placed into the subarachnoid space containing cerebrospinal fluid (CSF) surrounding the spinal cord.

spinal headache A headache caused by a small hole in the protective covering of the spinal cord (dura), resulting in a leak of the cushioning fluid (cerebrospinal fluid). It is usually brought on by sitting up and relieved with lying down. It is often caused when an epidural needle is inadvertently advanced too far.

standard monitors Devices connected to a patient that detect, interpret, and display bodily functions such as heart rate/rhythm, blood pressure, oxygen level, breathing rate, and temperature.

sterile Free from bacteria and viruses.

stretch receptors Nerve endings in the stomach that send signals to the brain that the stomach is too full.

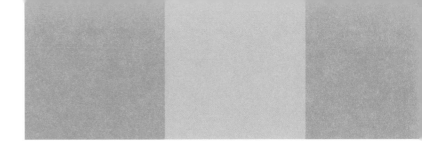

subarachnoid space The space between the arachnoid and pia matter-covering layers of the brain and spinal cord. It is filled with a body fluid called cerebrospinal fluid (CSF), which acts as a cushion for the brain and spinal cord.

surgeon A physician who operates.

surgeon-anesthetists Usually an oral/maxillofacial surgeon. Such specialists are also fully trained to administer anesthesia to a patient.

surgical consent form An agreement between the physician and patient to have an operation or procedure done. It includes an understanding of risks and benefits by the patient.

time out A verification among doctors and nurses that the correct procedure and site of surgery is being done on the right person.

topical anesthetics Creams and gels containing local anesthetic that can be applied to the skin.

total intravenous anesthesia (TIVA) A technique where all anesthetic agents are given through an intravenous line. No anesthetic gases are used.

toxicity Adverse effects resulting from high concentrations of a substance such as a local anesthetic.

transesophageal echocardiograph (TEE) A device that uses sound waves to take real-time pictures of the beating heart. A tube-like probe is placed through the mouth into the esophagus (food pipe). The tip of the probe sits behind the heart, sending off ultrasound waves. The waves bounce back off the heart and create a detailed picture of the heart chambers and what is happening inside the heart.

twilight sleep Light anesthesia without loss of consciousness. The condition relieves anxiety and may result in amnesia.

ventilation The exchange of air between the lungs and the atmosphere so that oxygen can be exchanged for carbon dioxide in the tiny air pockets in the lungs. *See also* mechanical ventilation.

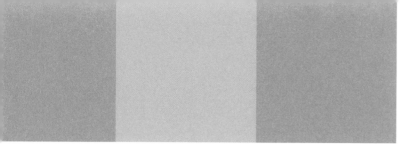

vertebrae The individual bones along the back protecting the spinal cord. There is a hole in the middle of each bone for the spinal cord to run through. The space between each bone is the site where spinal and epidural needles are placed.

vital signs The signs of life and body functions. These include heart rate, breathing rate, oxygen level, blood pressure, and temperature.

vomiting center A location in the brain that receives signals from different parts of the body such as sights, smells, mental thoughts, a full stomach, distasteful food, car motion, or chemicals in the blood. It then sends out signals throughout the body to coordinate the act of vomiting.

walking epidural A form of epidural anesthetic used in pregnant laboring patients. A low dose of local anesthetic and narcotic is given, resulting in pain relief but without numbness in the legs.

warming blanket A plastic blanket placed on a patient that is infused with warm air, much like a hair dryer blowing between two plastic sheets. The blanket can be placed over the chest and arms or from the waist down.

references

Chapter 1

Bahvsar J, Montgomery D, Li J, et al. Impact of duty hour restriction on quality of care and clinical outcomes. *American Journal of Medicine* 2007; 32(22): E649–E651.

Kuczkowski KM. Lifestyle changes in U.S. academic anesthesia: quo vadis? (letter). *Anesthesia and Analgesia* 2004; 99: 628–629.

Murray DJ, Boulet JR, Avidan M, et al. Performance of residents and anesthesiologists in a simulation-based skill assessment. *Anesthesiology* 2007; 107(5): 705–713.

Pino RM. The nature of anesthesia and procedural sedation outside the operating room. *Current Opinion in Anesthesiology* 2007; 20(4): 347–351.

Chapter 2

Chao D, Nanda A. Spinal epidural abscess: a diagnostic challenge. *American Family Physician* 2002; 65(7): 1341–1346.

Christie IW, McCabe S. Major complications of epidural analgesia after surgery: results of a six year survey. *Anaesthesia* 2007; 62(4): 335–341.

Cullen DJ, Bogdanov E, Htut N. Spinal epidural hematoma: occurrence in the absence of known risk factors: a case series. *Journal of Clinical Anesthesia* 2004; 16(5): 376–381.

Horlocker TT, Wedel DJ. Ultrasound guided regional anesthesia: in search of the holy grail. *Anesthesia and Analgesia* 2007; 104(5): 1009–1111.

Parker BM. Anesthesia and anesthesia techniques: impacts on perioperative management and postoperative outcomes. *Cleveland Clinic Journal of Medicine* 2006; 73(S1): S13–S17.

Stoelting RK, Miller RD. *Basics of Anesthesia* (5th ed.). Philadelphia: Churchill-Livingston, 2007.

Wang LP, Haurberg J, Schmidt JF. Incidence of spinal epidural abscess after epidural analgesia: a national 1 year survey. *Anesthesiology* 1999; 91(6): 1928–1936.

Chapter 3

American Society of Anesthesiologists Task Force on Preoperative Fasting. Practice guidelines for preoperative fasting and the use of pharmacologic agents to reduce the risk of pulmonary aspiration: application to healthy patients undergoing elective procedure. *Anesthesiology* 1999; 90(3): 896–905.

Ferschl MB, Tung A, Sweitzer B, et al. Preoperative clinic visits reduce operating room cancellations and delays. *Anesthesiology* 2005; 103(4): 855–859.

Chapter 4

Alfredsdottir H, Bjonsdottir K. Nursing and patient safety in the operating room. *Journal of Advanced Nursing* 2008; 61(1): 29–37.

Makary MA, Sexton JB, Freischlag JA, et al. Patient safety in surgery. *Annals of Surgery* 2006; 243(5): 628–635.

Undre S, Sevdalis N, Healey AN, et al. Teamwork in the operating theatre: cohesion or confusion? *Journal of Evaluation of Clinical Practice* 2006; 12(2): 182–189.

Chapter 5

Lake CL, Hines RL, Casey DB. *Clinical Monitoring: Practical Applications for Anesthesia and Critical Care.* Philadelphia: Saunders, 2001.

Thompson JP, Mahajan RP. Monitoring the monitors—beyond risk management. *British Journal of Anesthesia* 2006; 97(1): 1–3.

Chapter 6

Aldrete JA. The post anesthesia recovery score revisited. *Journal of Clinical Anesthesia* 1995; 7(1): 89–91.

American Society of Anesthesiologists Task Force on Postanesthetic Care. Practice guidelines for postanesthetic care. *Anesthesiology* 2002; 96: 742–752.

Chung F, Kayumov L, Sinclair DR, et al. What is the driving performance of ambulatory surgical patients after general anesthesia? *Anesthesiology* 2005; 103(5): 951–956.

Mattila K, Toivonen J, Janhunen L, et al. Postdischarge symptoms after ambulatory surgery: first-week incidence, intensity, and risk factors. *Anesthesia and Analgesia* 2005; 101: 1643–1650.

Chapter 7

Grass J. Patient-controlled analgesia. *Anesthesia and Analgesia* 2005; 101: S44–S61.

Helman C. *Culture, Health and Illness*. Bristol, UK: John Write and Sons, 1985.

Ilfeld BM, Wright TW, Enneking FK, et al. Total elbow arthroplasty as an outpatient procedure using a continuous infraclavicular nerve block at home: a prospective case report. *Regional Anesthesia and Pain Medicine* 2006; 31(2): 172–176.

Kim H, Dionne RA. Genetics, pain and analgesia. *Pain Clinical Updates* 2005; 13(3): 1–4.

May J, White HC, Leonard-White A, et al. The patient recovering from alcohol or drug addiction: special issues for the anesthesiologist. *Anesthesia and Analgesia* 2001; 92: 1601–1608.

Mitra S, Sinatra RS. Perioperative management of acute pain in the opioid dependent patient. *Anesthesiology* 2004; 101: 212–227.

O'Conner PG. Methods of detoxification and their role in treating patients with opioid dependence. *Journal of the American Medical Association* 2005; 294(8): 961–963.

Palos GR, Cantor SB, Aday LA, et al. Asking the community about cutpoints used to describe mild, moderate, and severe pain. *Journal of Pain* 2006; 7(1): 49–56.

Weingarten TN, Sprung J, Ackerman JD, et al. Anesthesia and patients with congenital hyposensitivity to pain. *Anesthesiology* 2006; 105(2): 338–345.

Chapter 8

Crockett RJ, Pruzinsky T, Persing JA. The influence of plastic surgery "Reality TV" on cosmetic surgery: patient expectations and decision making. *Plastic and Reconstructive Surgery* 2007; 120: 316–324.

Fleisher LA, Pasternak LR, Lyles A. A novel index of elevated risk of inpatient hospital admission immediately following outpatient surgery. *Archives of Surgery* 2007; 142: 263–268.

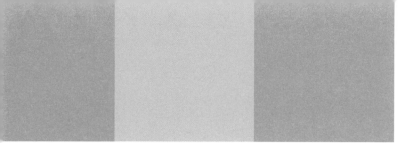

Haiken E. The making of the modern face. *Social Research* 2000; 67(1): 81–97.

Jakubietz M, Jakubietz RJ, Kloss DF, et al. Body dysmorphic disorder: diagnosis and approach. *Plastic and Reconstructive Surgery* 2007; 119(6): 1924–1930.

Mandal A, Imran A, McKinnell T, et al. Unplanned admissions following ambulatory plastic surgery: a retrospective study. *Annals of the Royal College of Surgeons of England* 2005; 87: 466–468.

Chapter 9

American Obesity Association Web site: www.obesity.org

Casati A, Putzu M. Anesthesia in the obese patient: pharmacokinetic considerations. *Journal of Clinical Anesthesia* 2005; 17(2): 134–145.

Ebert TJ, Shanker H, Haake RM. Perioperative considerations for patients with morbid obesity. *Anesthesiology Clinics* 2006; 24(3): 621–636.

Ezri T, Medalion B, Weisenberg M, et al. Increased body mass index per se is not a predictor of difficult laryngoscopy. *Canadian Journal of Anesthesia* 2003; 50(2): 179–183.

Juvin P, Lavaut E, Dupont H, et al. Difficult tracheal intubation is more common in obese than lean patients. *Anesthesia and Analgesia* 2003; 97: 595–600.

Mayo Clinic Web site: www.mayoclinic.com

Chapter 10

Chestnut DH. *Obstetric Anesthesia: Principles and Practice* (3rd ed.). St. Louis: Mosby, 2004.

Munnur U, de Boisblanc B, Suresh MS. Airway problems in pregnancy. *Critical Care Medicine* 2005; 33(10): S259–S268.

Wong CA, Scavone BM, Peaceman AM, et al. The risk of cesarean delivery with neuraxial analgesia given early versus late in labor. *New England Journal of Medicine* 2005; 352(7): 655–665.

Chapter 11

Costarino AT, Brenn BR. Pediatric anesthesiology. *Anesthesiology Clinics of North America* 2005; 23(4): 573–886.

Frank LS, Spencer C. Informing parents about anaesthesia for children's surgery: a critical literature review. *Patient Education and Counseling* 2005; 59: 117–125.

Hurford WE. *Clinical Procedures of the Massachusetts General Hospital* (6th ed.). Philadelphia: Lippincott Williams and Wilkins, 2002.

Chapter 12

Dionne RA, Yagiela JA, Cote CJ, et al. Balancing efficacy and safety in the use of oral sedation in dental outpatients. *Journal of the American Dental Association* 2006; 137: 502–513.

Dionne RA, Yagiela JA, Moore PA, et al. Comparing efficacy and safety of four intravenous sedation regimens in dental outpatients. *Journal of the American Dental Association* 2001; 132: 740–751.

Malamed SF, Gagnon S, Leblanc D, et al. Articaine hydrochloride: a study of the safety of a new amide local anesthetic. *Journal of the American Dental Association* 2001; 132: 177–185.

Ryding HA, Murphy HJ. Use of nitrous oxide and oxygen for conscious sedation to manage pain and anxiety. *Journal of the Canadian Dental Association* 2007; 73(8): 711–711d.

Steinkruger G, Nusstein J, Reader A, et al. The significance of needle bevel orientation in achieving a successful inferior alveolar nerve block. *Journal of the American Dental Association* 2006; 137: 1685–1691.

Chapter 13

Apfel CC, Kortilla K, Abdalla M, et al. A factorial trial of six interventions for the prevention of postoperative nausea and vomiting. *New England Journal of Medicine* 2004; 350 (24): 2441–2451.

Apfel CC, Laara E, Koivuranta M, et al. A simplified risk score for predicting postoperative nausea and vomiting. *Anesthesiology* 1999; 91: 693–700.

Eberhart LH, Geldner G, Kranke P, et al. The development and validation of a risk score to predict the probability of postoperative vomiting in pediatric patients. *Anesthesia and Analgesia* 2004; 99: 1630–1637.

Fetzer SJ, Hand MA, Bouchard PA, et al. Self-care activities for postdischarge nausea and vomiting. *Journal of Perianesthesia Nursing* 2005; 20(4): 249–254.

Gan TJ, Meyer T, Apfel CC, et al. Consensus guidelines for managing post-operative nausea and vomiting. *Anesthesia and Analgesia* 2003; 97: 62–71.

Chapter 14

American Society of Anesthesiologists Task Force on Intraoperative Awareness. Practice Advisory for Intra-operative Awareness and Brain Function Monitoring. *Anesthesiology* 2006; 104: 847–864.

Avidan MS, Zhang L, Burnside BA. Anesthesia awareness and the bispectral index. *New England Journal of Medicine* 2008; 358(11): 1097–1108.

Dahaba AA. Different conditions that could result in the bispectral index indicating an incorrect hypnotic state. *Anesthesia and Analgesia* 2005; 101: 765–773.

Joint Commission on Accreditation of Healthcare Organizations. Preventing, and managing the impact of anesthesia awareness. *Sentinel Event Alert* 2004; 32. Available at www.jcaho.org.

Myles PS, Leslie K, McNeil J, et al. Bispectral index monitoring to prevent awareness during anesthesia: the B-Aware randomized controlled trial. *Lancet* 2004; 363: 1757–1763.

Pollard RJ, Coyle JP, Gilbert RL, et al. Intraoperative awareness in a regional medical system: a review of 3 years' data. *Anesthesiology* 2007; 106(2): 269–274.

Rampersad SE, Mulroy M. A case of awareness despite an "adequate depth of anesthesia" as indicated by a bispectral index monitor. *Anesthesia and Analgesia* 2005; 100: 1363, 1364.

Sebel PS, Bowdle TA, Ghoneim MM, et al. The incidence of awareness during anesthesia: a multicenter United States study. *Anesthesia and Analgesia* 2004; 99: 833–839.

Spitellie PH, Megan A, Holmes MS, et al. Awareness during anesthesia. *Anesthesiology Clinics of North America* 2002 (20): 555–570.

Anesthesia through the Ages

Faulconer A, Keys T. *Foundations of Anesthesiology* (2 vols.). Park Ridge, IL: Wood Library-Museum of Anesthesiology, 1993.

Gordon BL. *Medicine throughout Antiquity*. Philadelphia: F. A. Davis, 1949.

Mettler C. *History of Medicine*. Philadelphia: Blakiston, 1947.

Sykes K; Bunker J (contrib. ed.). *Anaesthesia and the Practice of Medicine: Historical Perspectives*. London: Royal Society of Medicine Press, 2007.

index

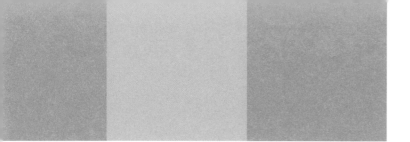

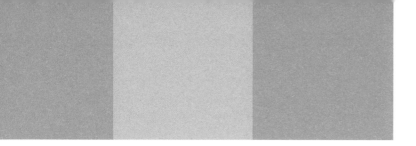

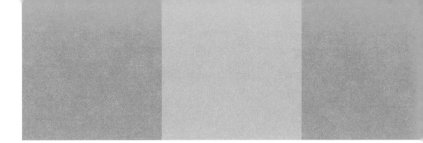

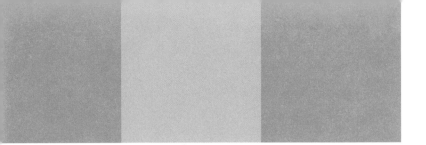

about the author

Panchali Dhar, MD, is assistant professor of clinical anesthesiology at New York-Presbyterian Hospital, Weill Medical College of Cornell University. She is board-certified in internal medicine and anesthesiology.

Dr. Dhar obtained her medical degree from New York University Medical School, where she also completed residencies in internal medicine and anesthesiology. She has also trained and worked at New York health-care institutions including New York University Langone Medical Center, Bellevue Hospital, and the Manhattan Veteran Affairs Hospital. She lives in New York City.